THE UV ADVANTAGE

Michael F. Holick, Ph.D., MD.

Professor of Medicine, Dermatology,
Physiology, and Biophysics
Boston University Medical Center

and Mark Jenkins

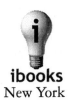

ibooks
New York

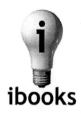

ibooks

1230 Park Avenue
New York, New York 10128
Tel: 212-427-7139 • Fax: 212-860-8852
bricktower@aol.com • www.BrickTowerPress.com

Library of Congress Cataloging-in-Publication Data
Holick, M.F. (Michael F.)
    The UV advantage : new medical breakthroughs reveal powerful health benefits
from sun exposure and tanning / Michael Holick and Mark Jenkins. – 2nd ed.
        p.   cm.
    Includes bibliographical references and index.
    ISBN 978-1-59687-900-3
    1. Solar radiation—Health aspects—Popular works. I. Jenkins, Mark.
II. Title: Ultraviolet advantage. [DNLM: 1. Sunlight—Popular Works.
2. Vitamin D—biosynthesis—Popular Works. QT 230 H732u 2003]
QP82.2.L5   H635
613'.193—dc21   2003002114

First Trade Paper Edition, April 2009

*Dedicated to the memory
of my good friend Don Christal,
who championed heliotherapy
and had a true appreciation
of the benefits of sunlight.*

CONTENTS

ACKNOWLEDGMENTS

This book would not have come into being without the involvement of many family members, friends and colleagues.

I am especially grateful to my wife Sally Ann and our children, Michael Todd and Emily Ann, for their support and understanding during the time-consuming process of creating a book of this complexity.

Thanks also to my coauthor Mark Jenkins, my literary agent Carol Mann, as well as all others who were involved in the "making" of this book.

Of course I am indebted to the numerous technicians, students, fellows, and colleagues with whom I have collaborated over the years in the field of photobiology. I am particularly appreciative of the assistance, counsel and inspiration given to me by Dr. John Adams, Dr. Mary Allen, Dr. George Brainard, Dr. Tai Chen, Dr. Farhad Chimeh, Dr. Thomas Clemens, Dr. Bess Dawson-Hughes, Sheila DeCastro, R.N., Dr. Hector DeLuca, Diane Digirolamo, R.N., Dr. Cerima Durokovic, Dr. Gary Ferguson, Drs. Cedric and Frank Garland, Dr. William Gehrmann, Dr. Barbara Gilchrest, Dr. William Grant, Ms. Nancy Hanafin, Dr. Robert Heaney, Mr. Daniel Jamieson, Dr. Ernst Jung, Dr. David Kenney, Dr. Douglas Kiel, Dr. Albert Kligman, Dr. Loren Kline, Dr. Polyxeni Koutkia, Dr. Rolfdieter Krause, Mona Lauture, R.N., Mr. Joe Levy, Dr. Clifford Lo, Dr. Zhiren Lu, Dr. Alan Malabanan, Dr. Trond Marksted, Mr. Jeffrey Mathieu, Dr. Lois Matsuoko, Dr. Carlos Mautalen, Ms. Julia McLaughlin, Janeen McNeil, R.N., Dr. Carolyn Moore, Barbara Nayak, R.N., Mr. John Overstreet, Dr. John Parrish, Dr. Ralf Paus, Dr. Alberto Perez, Mr. Kelly Persons, Dr. John Pettifor, Dr. John T. Potts, Jr., Dr. Rahul Ray, Mrs. Swapna Ray, Dr. Jorg Reichrath, Mr. Jack Reilly, Dr. Clifford Rosen, Mr. Matt Russell, Dr. Gary Schwartz, Mr. Jim Shepherd, Mrs. Elizabeth Southworth, Ms. Catherine St. Clair, Dr. Mark St. Lezin, Dr. Vin Tangpricha, Dr. Xiao Tian, Dr. Duane Ulrey, Dr. Ann Webb, Mr. Lyman Whitlatch, Mr. Frederic Wolff, Mr. Jörg Wolff, Dr. Jacobo Wortsman, Michele Wright-Nealand, Dr. Michael Young, and Dr. Susie Zanello.

PREFACE

IT HAPPENED AGAIN the other day. I was in a hotel elevator and overheard a woman telling her companion how much she loved to be in the sun but she couldn't anymore because "it would kill her." It's the kind of thing I hear all the time, and it is what inspired me to write this book.

My goal is to help put society's attitude toward sunlight into proper perspective. I've been researching this subject for many years, and institutions from NASA to the National Zoo have come to me for advice. I've successfully treated a variety of serious diseases with exposure to the kind of radiation that's in sunlight (UVB), including osteoporosis, osteomalacia, high blood pressure, and psoriasis. Results of my studies have been published in major scientific and medical journals.

Most people have taken my support of moderate sun exposure to mean I advocate *tanning*. Not true. Do I lie out in the sun for hours at a time or frequent tanning salons? *No.* Do I go out in strong sunshine without a sunscreen on, and does my skin get tanned? *Yes.* Why? Because I recognize that my body needs a certain amount of sun exposure to be healthy. Do I put sunscreen on after a certain amount of time? *Yes.* Why? Because I understand that there are risks as well as benefits associated with being in the sun. I recently ran into that poster boy for tanning, George Hamilton. When he found out I was an advocate of sun exposure, he jokingly commented that my skin was so pale he could see his reflection in it!

I am advocating *common sense*, something often in short supply in modern America's approach to health. I also respect your right to do something that may make you look and feel better. I believe I can help you make choices that will pursue this goal in a healthier, more effective way. Our society doesn't seem to believe in a happy medium, only in extremes. Do not be afraid—you are not going to die just because you go out in the sun. Indeed, the UVB radiation in sunlight is essential for good health. The notion that we have to protect ourselves from the sun all the time is misguided and unhealthy. This sun phobia explains why so many people are suffering from conditions related to sun deprivation.

Part of the problem is that our national health leaders have lost faith in the public's ability to make informed decisions about health. Their attitude seems to be: *We can't trust the public to be judicious in its attitude toward sun exposure, so let's tell people they shouldn't spend any time in the sun.* The problem with this presumptuous approach is that eliminating sun exposure is out-and-out *un*healthy. Lack of sunlight is associated with a host of conditions from colon, breast, prostate, and ovarian cancer to heart disease, high blood pressure, Type 1 diabetes, multiple sclerosis, and depression. Many of these policymakers are out of touch with new research and are unfamiliar with the growing body of evidence that shows how important sunlight is to human health.

Your overall well-being depends in part on developing an appropriate relationship with the sun. However, it can be a challenge to get the kind of information you need to establish such a relationship. The main purpose of this book is to provide you with an unbiased understanding of the issues at hand.

Equipped with this information, you will be able to make your own decision about what your relationship to the sun should be. You, too, can learn to use sunlight for health.

CHAPTER ONE

The Facts of Light

*Why you need sunlight,
and how you got conned into
thinking it was bad for you*

I T WAS THE SUMMER of 1997 and for months my staff and I had been studying the vitamin D status of a random group of people living in the Boston area. As Director of the General Clinical Research Center and Professor of Medicine, Dermatology, Physiology, and Biophysics at Boston University Medical Center, I had designed and was leading this study. I was sitting in my office when the results came in. Although I had a strong suspicion by that time of what the study would reveal, the actual numbers were staggering. Fully 42 percent of the people we studied were vitamin D deficient. My study, which was accepted for publication in *Lancet* (only one in a hundred papers submitted to this renowned journal are published), confirmed what most scientists in the field believe. That is, there is an epidemic of vitamin D deficiency in the United States and much of the Western world. Some have called this a "silent epidemic" because, although the consequences of vitamin D deficiency are profound, there are often no obvious symptoms.

What is the cause of this "silent epidemic"? In part, it is the result of very few people these days eating enough foods rich in vitamin D—mostly "oily" fish such as salmon and mackerel. Also, most Americans do not compensate for a diet poor in vitamin D by following recommendations to drink enough vitamin D-fortified milk or to take nutritional supplements. (Milk usually contains far less vitamin D than the FDA approves of.)

Still, none of these factors is as important in explaining the widespread levels of vitamin D deficiency as is the fact that as a society we are increasingly choosing to deprive ourselves of our most important source of vitamin D—sunlight.

Exaggerated warnings about the perils of sun exposure are driving Americans to hide beneath long sleeves, floppy hats, and wraparound sunglasses and to slather every square inch of skin that isn't covered with high-SPF sunscreens. (My studies have shown that SPF 8 reduces vitamin D production by 97.5 percent and SPF 15 reduces it by 99.9 percent). The result of all this is to block out the sun that humans need to make vitamin D. The inescapable fact is that humans have evolved in such a way as to be dependant on sunshine for life and health. Sunlight is the fuel that enables your body to manufacture vitamin D. When you block out sunlight with sunscreens and head-to-toe clothing, you stop that supply of fuel and your body can't make enough vitamin D.

Why does this matter? The short answer is that the benefits of vitamin D on human health are many, varied, and profound. We'll take a thorough look at these benefits in chapter 4. Suffice it to say that in some respected medical circles, sunlight is being described as a "wonder drug." It can provide "immu-

How Sun Exposure Benefits Human Health

- Improves bone health
- Enhances mental health (SAD, PMS, depression, general mood)
- Prevents certain cancers
- Improves heart health
- Alleviates skin disorders
- Decreases risk of autoimmune disorders, including multiple sclerosis, Type 1 diabetes mellitus, and rheumatoid arthritis
- Alleviates conditions related to obesity that prevent participation in an exercise program

nity" against some of the most devastating diseases around, including heart attack, stroke, osteoporosis, and certain of the most deadly internal cancers. The statistics speak volumes. Some researchers, notably Dr. William Grant, have proven that, in America, increased sun exposure would result in 185,000 fewer cases of internal cancers every year and 30,000 fewer deaths (specifically cancers of the breast, ovaries, colon, prostate, bladder, uterus, esophagus, rectum, and stomach). Sunlight has a similarly dramatic effect on high blood pressure, one of the leading causes of heart attack and stroke—people who spend time in the sun or on a tanning bed experience a blood pressure–lowering effect similar to that of standard medications that have unpleasant side effects. We've found that sunlight has a beneficial effect on heart health equal to exercise. Then there's bone health. Sun exposure helps build and maintain bone density and reduces fractures, one of the main causes of death and disability among senior citizens. Humans also need sunlight to control the biological clocks that regulate mood, and appropriate sun exposure is responsible for keeping down rates of depression associated with seasonal affective disorder (SAD) and premenstrual syndrome (PMS). Let's not forget that sunlight plain old makes you feel better—not something to be dismissed in this high-stress world in which many of us live.

Those who heed warnings to avoid the sun because "sunlight is dangerous" (whom I refer to as "sun-phobes") are robbed of the life-sustaining benefits of sun exposure—and this idea denies basic evolutionary science.

In the Beginning . . .

From the beginning of recorded time, humans have worshipped the sun for its therapeutic properties. This can be seen in cave paintings that show that exposure to sunlight was necessary for life and good health. Medical practitioners reported the benefits of sun exposure on heart health 6,000 years ago in the time of the ancient Egyptian pharaohs Ramses and Akhenaten. Sun therapy was also praised by the legendary Hippocrates (creator of the Hippocratic Oath) and the doctors of bygone Rome and Arabia. The Egyptians, Mesopotamians, and Greeks all had sun deities, and the influence of the sun in religious belief also appears in Zoroastrianism, Mithraism, Roman religion, Hinduism, Buddhism, and among the Druids of England, the Aztecs of Mexico, the Incas of Peru, and many Native American groups.

That ancient peoples instinctively understood that sunshine was good for them is not surprising. Humans have depended on sunlight to sustain life and health since our ancestors slithered out of the primordial ooze. Without the calcium-rich environment of the bubbling saline oceans in which life evolved—and from which we could absorb calcium right into our primitive skeletons—our creepy-crawling ancestors got their calcium on land by eating plants. The main job of calcium is to build bones, and these ancient relatives of ours developed a system of absorbing the calcium through diet into the bones. This chemical process required the presence of vitamin D, which was made in the skin when it was exposed to sunlight.

Fast-forward a couple million years, and Homo sapiens were still using sunlight to make the vitamin D needed to regulate the calcium necessary for bone health. Early humans lived near the equator where sunlight is plentiful, and they developed dark, melanin-rich skins that protected them against sunburn but still "let in" enough sunlight to make vitamin D. As humans started to migrate away from the equator to regions where sunlight is less intense, and where for several months of the year the sun isn't strong enough for the human body to make vitamin D, skin got less pigmented so it would more effectively "let in" the sun when it was available. The farther north humans migrated, the fairer their skin became to make use of available sunlight. Eventually humans couldn't migrate any farther north because there wasn't enough sun to make the vitamin D needed to survive. Then something fascinating happened—humans developed the means to harvest the seas for vitamin D-rich fish and mammals of the sort still traditionally eaten by Eskimos and Scandinavians and that enable people to live in climates with very little sunlight.

Even today, people with fair skin don't require much exposure to sunlight to make enough vitamin D to be healthy, and people with dark skin are naturally well protected against sunburn. Conversely, people with fair skin get sunburned quite easily and may be susceptible to skin cancer, whereas dark-complected people more easily become vitamin D deficient when living in northern climates.

Although this is a very simplistic explanation for why humans need sunlight for health and life, it should put to rest the notion that sunlight is something humans must fear. Sunlight is necessary for human survival!

Sunlight 101

To fully understand the pros and cons of sun exposure, you need to know what's going on "up there" and how it affects you "down here."

Sunlight consists of a mixture of electromagnetic radiation of various wavelengths, from the longest, called infrared, through red, orange, yellow, green, blue, indigo and violet, to the shortest in wavelength, called ultraviolet (see figure 1.1).

Ultraviolet, or UV radiation, consists of UVA, UVB, and UVC. UVC is completely absorbed by the atmosphere. UVA and UVB reach earth's surface but have different effects on your body. UVA radiation causes wrinkles and in extremely high doses may be responsible for melanomas.

UVB is the form of radiation that reddens skin and that may be responsible, over the long term, for non-melanoma skin cancer. When UVB causes sunburns, it may contribute to

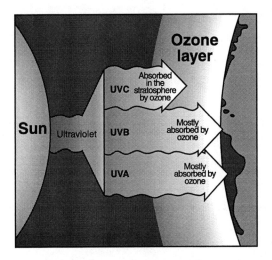

Figure 1.1 The sun produces electromagnetic
radiation of various wavelengths, including ultraviolet
A, B, and C.

melanoma. UVB is also the form of radiation that starts the reaction in skin that stimulates the production of vitamin D.

Until recently, most sunscreens only blocked UVB radiation, which may have precipitated the rise of melanoma in the
United States and other Western cultures. That's because sunscreens that block out only the burning UVB radiation enable
people to stay out in the sun for unlimited periods of time during which they are not protected against UVA radiation. Without any sunscreen at all, people would not have been able to
stay out in the sun long enough to receive the dosage of UVA
necessary to cause melanoma.

Thankfully, researchers have now developed "broad spectrum" sunscreens, which protect against both UVA and UVB
radiation.

The level of UV radiation that reaches the earth varies depending on several factors, including the following:

- **Stratospheric ozone.** The ozone layer absorbs most of the sun's radiation, but how much it absorbs depends on what time of year it is and certain other natural phenomena. As a whole, the ozone layer has thinned due to industrial pollution and now-banned substances previously emitted by refrigerants and certain consumer products such as hairspray.

- **Time of day.** UV levels are at their most intense at noontime, when the sun is at its highest point in the sky. When the sun is at its highest point, the UV radiation has the least distance to travel through the atmosphere to earth. Contrarily, the sun's radiation must pass through the atmosphere at a greater angle during the early morning and late afternoon, and therefore UV intensity is greatly diminished at those times.

- **Time of year.** The angle of the sun changes with the seasons. This causes the intensity of the UV radiation to vary as well. UV intensity is greatest during the summer months.

- **Latitude.** The sun's radiation is most intense at the equator where the sun is directly overhead and the radiation from it has to travel the shortest distance through the earth's ozone atmosphere. Therefore, at the equator, more UV radiation reaches the earth's surface from the sun. At higher latitudes, the sun is lower in the sky and

UV radiation has to travel a greater distance through thicker ozone to reach the earth's surface. This makes the UV radiation in middle and high latitudes less intense.

- **Altitude.** UV radiation is more intense at higher altitudes because there is less atmosphere to absorb it. When you are at higher altitudes, therefore, you are at greater risk of overexposure.

- **Weather conditions.** The more clouds there are, the less UV radiation can penetrate to the earth's surface. However, UV can still penetrate cloud cover, which explains why you can still get sunburned on a hazy summer's day.

- **Reflection.** Certain surfaces reflect UV radiation and increase its intensity even in shaded areas. Such surfaces include snow, sand, or water.

Science and Sunlight

When modern science began investigating the connection between sunlight and health, it was initially believed that the health benefits of sunlight were the result of the warmth generated by the sun. It was Sir Everhard Home, in the late 1700s and early 1800s, who deduced that it wasn't the heat of the sun's radiation but rather the occurrence of a chemical effect on the body caused by the sun that produced sunburn. Home also showed that dark-skinned people had a natural resistance to sunburn. In the 1820s, a Polish doctor named Jedrzej Sniadecki first observed that children who lived in the city of Warsaw had a much higher prevalence of rickets than youngsters who lived in the Polish countryside. Dr. Sniadecki thought it was probably the lack of sunshine in the cramped confines of Warsaw that was to blame for this widespread condition. Sniadecki was able to successfully treat the afflicted city kids by taking them into the countryside for sun exposure, which began a long-standing tradition for treating this condition. Floating Hospital in Boston, now a modern multistoried structure, got its name because it was originally a large boat that, in the summertime, took children with rickets into Boston Harbor to be bathed in sunshine. Although the exact relationship between sunlight and bone development was not yet understood, a health movement was pioneered by Arnold Rikli at the end of the 1800s with this motto: "Water works wonders, air can do even more, but light works best of all."

By the beginning of the twentieth century, scientists had determined that it was the UV radiation in sunlight that stimulated the production of vitamin D in the human body. They determined that this was important for a variety of health reasons. Based on findings that the vitamin D created by sun exposure improved bone health, the dairy industries of Europe and the United States started fortifying milk with vitamin D. A craze was under way, and vitamin D fortification was being touted by the manufacturers of products as varied as Bond Bread, Rickter's Hot Dogs, Twang Soda, and even Schlitz Beer.

The first few decades of the twentieth century were the heyday of photobiology and heliotherapy. Photobiology is a branch of science that investigates the effect of natural and artificial radiation on all life forms; heliotherapy focuses on the sun's abilities to heal the sick. Photobiologists and heliotherapists were credited with developing effective treatments for rickets, tuberculosis, and psoriasis. Hospitals all over Europe and the United States had built solariums and balconies so they could offer their patients a pleasant place to enjoy the sun's healing rays. In addition, a photobiologist had won the Nobel Prize for Medicine. However, the tide was about to change.

Frightening People Out of the Daylight

So what happened? How did we reach a point in our history when sun became something to be feared instead of worshipped? Shunned instead of desired? The simple answer lies in the fact that there are many billions of dollars to be made in emphasizing the only major medical downside of sun exposure (non-melanoma skin cancer) and not much money to be made in promoting the sun's many benefits.

Medicine has long known that, despite all the sun's benefits, a health downside of sun exposure is non-melanoma skin cancer. In the 1920s, it was recognized that farmers in Europe developed skin cancer on their most sun-exposed areas—their ears, face, nose, and backs of their hands. In 1941, the first issue of the *Journal of Cancer* put the issue in perfect perspective, stating that an increased risk of non-melanoma skin cancer was one of the prices to be paid for a decreased risk of cancer of the prostate, breast, and colon. Unfortunately, in the past quarter century, the relationship between sunlight and skin cancer has been blown out of proportion. The major culprits are the cosmetic wing of the pharmaceutical industry and some dermatologists.

Pharmacology Takes Over

The decline of sunlight as a popular and successful treatment for a variety of diseases was hastened by major medical breakthroughs. It started with the discovery of penicillin in 1928. The success of this and other wonder drugs heralded the beginning of the era of pharmacology and saved the lives of millions. However, it also precipitated the eclipse of disciplines such as heliotherapy and photobiology, which appeared quaint and outdated by comparison. It wasn't long before people had been converted en masse to the idea that synthetic drugs were much more effective in preventing and curing most maladies that affect humankind than anything Mother Nature had to offer—a belief that largely prevails today.

In the 1960s and 1970s, as the leisure culture expanded and people were spending more time outdoors, the "cosme-ceutical" industry developed anti-sunburn creams that gave the user a false sense of security and encouraged excessive sun exposure. These products began making extraordinary amounts of money for the companies. Although the products were initially introduced to prevent sunburn, they soon were being cannily marketed to prevent skin cancer. There is an important role for modern sunscreens in preventing skin cancer, and people should control sun exposure in the same way they watch how much salt, sugar, and fat they eat and how much alcohol they drink. However, the sophisticated and aggressive "educational" campaigns funded by the cosme-ceutical industry have created an anti-sunshine hysteria that is detrimental to our health because it converts people into sun-phobes by convincing them that no amount of sun exposure is safe.

So desperate is the anti-sun lobby to convince you of the dangers of the sun so that you will buy its products year-round, its representatives will tell you with a straight face that if it's February in Boston and you're planning to walk to the corner store to buy a quart of milk or sit outside on your lunch break, you should wear sunscreen. This is wrong-headed and alarmist. Even on the sunniest February day, the sun isn't strong enough in New England or New York to increase your risk of skin cancer significantly. This is but one example of the kinds of inaccurate information the anti-sun lobby puts out to alarm people. In so doing, it convinces people of the need for its products and services.

The scare tactics of the cosme-ceutical industry have been embraced by most of the dermatology profession. These groups have worked in concert and have frightened the day-lights out of people—or, to put it more accurately, frightened people out of the daylight. It has turned them into sun-phobes.

To put the dangers of skin cancer in context, it's worthwhile looking at some statistics. Non-melanoma skin cancer, which may be caused by long-term sun exposure, has an extremely low death rate. Fewer than half of 1 percent of people who de-velop non-melanoma skin cancer die; non-melanoma skin can-cer claims 1,200 lives a year in the United States. Compare that with diseases that can be prevented by regular sun exposure. Colon and breast cancers, which may be prevented by regular sun exposure, have mortality rates of 20 to 65 percent and kill 138,000 Americans annually. Osteoporosis, a bone disease that can be mitigated by regular sun exposure, is endemic, affecting

25 million Americans. Every year, 1.5 million Americans with osteoporosis suffer bone fractures, which can be fatal when the person is elderly. Non-melanoma skin cancer is not something to be taken lightly, and I would never minimize its effects on sufferers, but in public health terms, it is relatively unimportant when compared with a host of killer diseases that can be prevented by regular, moderate sun exposure.

What about melanoma? This is an important question. Though rare, melanomas are by far the most dangerous form of skin cancer, and, if left untreated, they are often fatal. Eighty percent of all skin cancer fatalities are attributed to this type of cancer. However—and this is a critical point—there is no credible scientific evidence that moderate sun exposure causes melanomas. In chapter 2, I will clear up the confusion surrounding the relationship between sun exposure and skin cancer, confusion that the media doesn't seem able to unravel and the anti-sun lobby has a vested interest in maintaining.

The anti-sun lobby also plays on people's fear of developing wrinkles—a growing concern in our youth-obsessed culture. It's true that sun exposure causes the skin to age prematurely, but it is possible to take advantage of the benefits of sun exposure while minimizing wrinkles. Interestingly, the type of sunscreens used in the 1960s probably predisposed people who sunbathed during that era to wrinkles. I'll take a closer look at this issue in chapter 3.

So why has no one stood up to the anti-sun lobby and said, "Hey, wait a minute, for too long you've exaggerated the dangers of sun exposure and ignored the fact that human beings need sunlight to live"? Well, I have! The problem is, whenever anyone challenges the anti-sun coalition doctrine that sun exposure does nothing but cause skin cancer and wrinkles—usually by publishing a new study that demonstrates a positive link between sunlight and disease prevention—this news is drowned out by another well-funded round of disinformation about the hazards of sun exposure. The bibliography at the end of the book lists many of the published studies that show the beneficial association between the vitamin D you get from sunlight and many areas of health.

It's difficult to get the facts out because there is no sun lobby. Sunshine is free, after all, so there's not much money to be made extolling its virtues. The indoor tanning industry has tried to step up to the plate (modern indoor tanning equipment provides many of the same benefits as natural sun exposure). However, the indoor tanning industry consists of numerous small, independent companies that could hardly be considered unified. The industry's trade organization, the Indoor Tanning Association, is a pauper compared with the wealthy princes representing the cosme-ceutical industry and the dermatology profession, and it has trouble making itself heard over the anti-sun din.

It doesn't help that media outlets have little appetite for "feel good" health stories—they believe their readers are more engaged by stories about what's going to kill them rather than what will make them feel better. Of course, it's also important to understand that newspaper editors and TV producers are busy men and women. When slickly packaged information about the "hazards of sun exposure" lands on their desks and no one contests this information, they are inclined to publish it verbatim to fill column inches and airtime. Often the "educational" material put out by the anti-sun lobby has been endorsed by eminent-sounding professionals and organizations.

Increasing numbers of studies are confirming the link between vitamin D and good health, however, and attitudes are beginning to change. More important, in the past few years there has been a breakthrough in our understanding of why sun exposure benefits health in so many ways, something that was not fully comprehended until recently. This breakthrough has forced people to take a closer look at the benefits of sun exposure. I am proud to say that I have been at the forefront of this research.

Sunshine and Cellular Health

I've been interested in the importance of vitamin D to human health for three decades. Way back in 1970, when I was a graduate student at the University of Wisconsin studying under the academic luminary Dr. Hector DeLuca, I isolated and identified the active form of vitamin D (1,25-dihydroxyvitamin D_3 [1,25$(OH)_2D_3$]) that provides the human body with so many health benefits. The immediate significance of this discovery was that doctors were able to prescribe tiny amounts of this substance to people whose bodies could not make their own active vitamin D due to kidney failure and who suffered severe bone problems as a result.

Even after all these years, I still find this area of science fascinating! I continue to perform studies and have published more than 200 research papers in peer-reviewed medical journals, which means the articles have to be approved by a screening board made up of experts in that particular field. Some of the journals that have published my studies include the *New England Journal of Medicine, Lancet,* and *Science.*

Medicine has long known that there is a clear and undisputed relationship between sun exposure and bone health. Without the vitamin D that comes almost entirely from the sun, your bones could not obtain the calcium they need to be strong. The pediatric bone disease rickets is unknown in children who get enough sun exposure, and, indeed, one of the most effective ways of treating kids with rickets is to get them into the sunshine.

The relationship between sun exposure and bone health is so incontrovertible that even the anti-sun lobby hems and haws about this issue. When its spokespeople are put on the spot, they usually mumble something along the lines of, "Kids gotta drink more milk." In fact, vitamin D-fortified milk was introduced to combat rickets, but much of the milk sold that is supposed to be rich in vitamin D does not actually contain the vitamin D it is supposed to. My own studies, published in the *New England Journal of Medicine,* proved this, and that research has been backed by other studies, including one by the Food and Drug Administration (FDA).

Rickets is again on the rise in our society—a shocking development given the medical advances during the past century. The main reason is that mothers breast-feed their children without taking a vitamin D supplement or providing their infants with any form of vitamin D supplementation. Human milk contains hardly any vitamin D, and without sun exposure or a vitamin D supplement, infants are at a high risk of developing rickets. Another reason rickets is being seen with increas-

Obesity: The Vitamin D Connection

Obesity and the vitamin D deficiency–related condition osteomalacia often go hand in hand. Osteomalacia is characterized by extreme bone and muscle pain and weakness. Being overweight predisposes a person to osteomalacia because the excess fat absorbs and holds onto the vitamin D from the sun and diet so that it cannot be used for bone building and cellular health. In addition, obese people are frequently vitamin D deprived because they go outside much less for practical and self-esteem-related reasons. A vicious cycle then begins.

When an obese person has osteomalacia, the bone and muscle pain and weakness make it virtually impossible to participate in any sort of physical activity that might help the individual manage his or her weight. As a result, the individual will become even more obese, which will in turn worsen his or her vitamin D status and exacerbate the osteomalacia.

Treating a person's vitamin D deficiency will cure osteomalacia and make it possible for the individual to exercise. A study I participated in showed that it was possible to increase obese people's vitamin D levels by exposing them to UVB radiation, in this case from tanning beds.

Treating obese people who have vitamin D deficiency–related osteomalacia may have benefits other than enabling them to exercise. Recent research has shown that being vitamin D deficient interferes with the secretion of a hormone called *leptin*, which signals the brain when a person has consumed enough fat. Building the vitamin D in that person's bloodstream to normal levels will restore that process.

Much more research needs to be done, but I think there is enormous potential for UVB exposure from the sun or artificial sources to be used to treat people with obesity.

ing frequency is that many kids these days spend too much time indoors and out of the sun or are slathered in sunscreen and made to wear protective clothing before they go out to play.

Increasing numbers of adults are developing a vitamin D deficiency–related bone condition known as osteomalacia (pronounced os-tee-oh-muh-LAY-shuh), sometimes called "adult rickets." This condition, characterized by vague bone and muscles aches, is frequently misdiagnosed as fibromyalgia or arthritis. The "fibromyalgia epidemic" that some doctors refer to may actually be a massive increase in vitamin D deficiency–related osteomalacia (see chapter 4 for more on this important subject).

We know that sunlight is essential for bone health, and we have understood this for more than a century. More recently, scientists have become interested in the fact that people living in sunny climates have a lower incidence of organ- and cellular-related conditions, such as heart disease and cancers of the breast, colon, ovaries, and prostate. Unlike the connection between sun exposure and bone health, the link between sun exposure and cellular and organ health was more difficult to establish. In part this is because much of what we now know is based on putting together research findings from different parts of the world, which was not possible in previous eras. Because it took longer for scientists to make the connection between sun exposure and cellular health, we only recently established what the connection actually is.

It's quite complicated, so before I get into that, let's back up to what was believed just fifteen years ago.

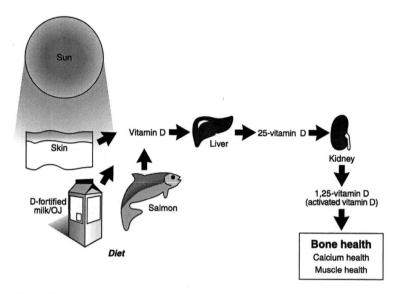

Figure 1.2 *Previous understanding of how vitamin D benefits health.* Until recently it was believed that the only place activated vitamin D (1,25[OH]₂D₃) could be made was in the kidneys from where it was disbursed in order to promote bone health.

Until the mid-1990s, it was believed that the kidneys make the body's entire supply of activated vitamin D (the only form of vitamin D that provides humans with health benefits). The kidneys make this supply from the 25-vitamin D in the bloodstream (25-hydroxyvitamin D, or $25[OH]D_3$) that is created by the liver out of the vitamin D that is made in the skin after sun exposure and, to a lesser extent, from foods that contain vitamin D (see figure 1.2). The supply of activated vitamin D that the kidneys actually manufacture is very small, and this supply doesn't change no matter how much 25-vitamin D there is in the bloodstream. In other words, you could dramatically increase the 25-vitamin D content in your bloodstream by lying on the beach all summer long, drinking quarts of milk, and eating mackerel at every meal, but your kidneys would still produce the same tiny trickle of activated vitamin D. The main job of this precious little amount of activated vitamin D, it was thought, was to contribute to bone health.

As the person who actually discovered the activated form of vitamin D, I was very closely involved with what was happening in the field of vitamin D research, and I have to be honest—there was something that was really bugging me!

Here's what we couldn't figure out. In response to increased exposure to sunlight, cellular and organ health benefits were occurring that appeared to be the work of activated vitamin D. These benefits included lower blood pressure and decreased risk of cancer. However, this couldn't be the work of activated vitamin D if what we believed we knew about the kidneys' production of activated vitamin D was true. There was apparently a connection between sun exposure and cellular and organ health. But our limited understanding of how activated vitamin D is produced prevented us from making the claim that one was responsible for the other.

All the while, we were teetering on the verge of a breakthrough in our understanding of the relationship between sunlight and cellular health. Finally, it happened. What my colleagues and I discovered in studies at the Vitamin D, Skin, and Bone Research Laboratory at Boston University Medical Center was that humans have the ability to make activated vitamin D throughout the body.

The process is extraordinary. Whereas once we thought that only the kidneys could activate vitamin D, we now understand that a variety of cells have this ability, including the

---

Could You Be Vitamin D Deficient?

You may be deficient in this vital vitamin if you:

- Rarely go out in the sun
- Always wear makeup and/or sunscreen on all exposed areas when outdoors
- Do not take a multivitamin
- Do not take a vitamin D supplement
- Do not eat a vitamin D–rich diet (oily fish, fish, liver, egg yolks, and so forth)
- Have dark skin and do not live near the equator
- Are older than 60 and live in a high latitude or deliberately avoid the sun

---

breast, prostate, colon, brain, skin, and probably most other tissues and cells. When the 25-vitamin D reaches and enters these cells, it is converted into activated vitamin D. Unlike the kidneys, however, which make activated vitamin D from 25-vitamin D and send it out through the bloodstream to the intestine and bones, in these cells 25-vitamin D is converted into activated vitamin D and used on the spot within the cell group (see figure 1.3). After it performs its important functions in the cell, the activated vitamin D extinguishes itself (that way it cannot leave the cell and enter the bloodstream to create a harmful form of vitamin D toxicity). Because this vitamin D activation process begins and ends within the cell, there is no evidence of increased activated vitamin D in the bloodstream, not even when more activated vitamin D is being made by

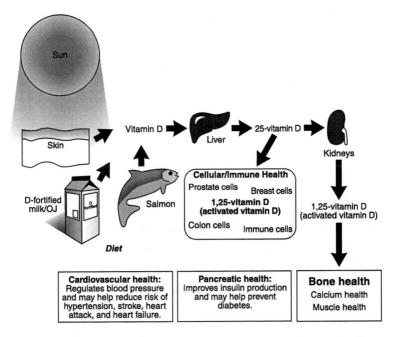

Figure 1.3 *New understanding of how vitamin D benefits health.* Recent break-through discoveries have shown that vitamin D can be activated within a variety of cells, including those of the prostate, breast, and colon, where it prevents the unhealthy cell proliferation characteristic of cancer. This process is self-contained within these cells. After the cells use the activated vitamin D, it is extinguished.

these cells. It is for this reason that scientists had difficulty making a connection between sun exposure and vitamin D.

This discovery is significant because we now know for sure that increasing vitamin D levels in our bloodstream via sun exposure, and to a lesser extent diet, will help lower the risk of several diseases—especially those caused by abnormal cell growth, such as cancer. We have also since discovered that our immune system has the ability to make activated vitamin D, meaning that sun exposure may have a role in preventing and treating autoimmune diseases such as multiple sclerosis, rheumatoid arthritis, and Type 1 diabetes.

My laboratory studies confirmed that activated vitamin D is an extremely potent substance that is one of the most effective inhibitors of abnormal cell growth. The discovery by my laboratory and other laboratories that cells throughout the body can activate vitamin D is a major breakthrough in vitamin D research. It is what's behind the emergent realization that—contrary to what we hear so often—the advantages of sun exposure far outweigh the potential negative consequences.

Add to this the growing body of research showing that sun exposure helps regulate circadian rhythms, thus preventing mood-related conditions such as seasonal affective disorder, premenstrual tension, and depression (see chapter 5). Some of the most exciting work in this area was done by me and my colleagues here in Boston. For example, we recently confirmed something that scientists had discovered in the 1980s that had never been followed up on: It's not just the brain that makes the "feel good" substance beta endorphin. When exposed to ultraviolet radiation, skin also makes beta endorphins. This may explain why people often feel so good after spending time at the beach or even in a tanning bed.

Why the Elderly and People of African Descent Need to Be Especially Concerned

The connections among sun exposure, vitamin D production, and disease prevention are important information for all of us, but they have special implications for two groups: older people and people of African descent. These two groups have a harder time making vitamin D than the rest of us.

The Elderly The older you get, the more difficult it is for your body to convert sun exposure into vitamin D. That means to maintain healthy levels of vitamin D in your body, you need more sun or you need to expose more skin area to sunlight. Unfortunately, older people are especially receptive to the alarmist warnings about excessive sun exposure. The elderly often decrease their sun exposure at a time when they need more of it to be healthy. Studies I have participated in have shown that well over half of Americans age 65 and older are vitamin D deficient. If you are a senior citizen, you need to be much more concerned about the risk of fracturing a hip because you are vitamin D deficient than the risk of getting wrinkles or skin cancer. Consider this alarming statistic: Approximately 300,000 hip fractures will occur in elderly men and women this year; 20 percent of those people will die within a year, and 50 percent will never regain mobility and have to move to a nursing home. For this population, the best advice is this: Get out in the sun! It's good for you.

People of African Descent People whose ancestors came from Africa and other countries near the equator have skin that evolved to be resistant to the sun's radiation. That this kind of skin is not efficient at converting the sun's radiation into vitamin D isn't an issue in Africa because there are unlimited amounts of sunshine on that continent. However, when people of African descent live in northern latitudes, they often become vitamin D deficient because their superprotective skin might not convert enough of the weaker, more limited amounts of sun into vitamin D. Studies I have participated in show that up to 80 percent of elderly African Americans are vitamin D deficient. What is remarkable is that the Centers for Disease Control has recently reported that 42 percent of African American women of childbearing age (15 to 49 years old) throughout the entire United States are vitamin D deficient by the end of winter. On average, 40 to 60 percent of African American adults are vitamin D deficient. African Americans are at increased risk of a variety of conditions associated with vitamin D deficiency, including cancer of the breast and prostate. Americans of African genetic lineage are also more likely to have forms of high blood pressure/hypertension and heart disease that are more resistant to drug treatment. Again, the best advice is simple—increase your exposure to sunlight.

Putting Sun Exposure into Perspective

Sun is crucial to your overall physical and mental well-being. Depending on what kind of skin you have, where you live, and what time of year it is, you need sun exposure in varying amounts to maintain adequate levels of vitamin D. It is true that there are some drawbacks to excessive sun exposure, and I examine these in depth in later chapters of this book. However, as you will see, the drawbacks of sun exposure pale in comparison with the health benefits.

Let's put the pros and cons of sunlight into perspective with an analogy. Exercise is another example of something that has both benefits and drawbacks but that is, on the whole, good for you. Everyone knows that exercising is good. It prevents a variety of chronic illnesses and makes you look and feel better. But if you exercise too much, or if you have certain predisposing risk factors—flat feet or a faulty backhand—then you may develop overuse conditions such as Achilles tendonitis or lateral epicondylitis ("tennis elbow"). Every year, people die of heart attacks while running or lifting weights. Nevertheless, no self-respecting doctor would take the position that "exercise is unhealthy." Most doctors will tell you to take certain precautions when exercising, but none would ever advise you not to be active.

The same goes for sun exposure. Sunlight is not "unhealthy." Precautions do need to be taken, but a regular, moderate amount of unprotected sun exposure is absolutely necessary for good health—as you will come to discover as you turn the pages of this book.

CHAPTER TWO

The Facts About Skin Cancer and Sunshine

Why the statement "sunlight causes cancer" is overstated, and how to harness the sun for health

FEW WORDS STRIKE FEAR in our hearts more than "cancer." Some people can't even bear to utter the term and instead substitute the phrase "the 'C' word." Fear of skin cancer is one of the main reasons for the hysteria over sun exposure. Thanks to how the cosmetic and pharmaceutical industries and some dermatologists have shaped people's attitudes through the media, the belief is that "Cancer kills, and sunshine causes cancer, so I'm going to avoid sunshine."

As is the case with so many supposed health axioms, the relationship between sunshine and cancer isn't as straightforward as most people think. There are a number of myths associated with what causes skin cancer. Before I set the record straight about the link between sun exposure and skin cancer, let's talk about the focus of all the attention—your skin.

Introducing Your Skin

You know that joke children play on each other? One wiseacre says to an unsuspecting friend, "Hey, your epidermis is showing!" You may remember as a kid wondering, "What is he talking about? Can everyone see my underwear or something?" That little prank was many people's introduction to their skin. As you discovered (to your great relief) when the joke was revealed, your epidermis is your skin, or, more accurately, the outer layer of your skin.

That everyone can see your skin is just one indication of how important it is. It is your body's largest organ and weighs about six pounds. Skin provides a protective covering for your entire body and protects you from sunlight, heat and cold, infections, toxins, and injury. Other important functions of the skin are that it regulates body temperature and retains water. And, of course, your skin helps you convert sunshine into vitamin D.

Your skin has two layers, the outer *epidermis* and the inner *dermis*. These two layers are quite different (see figure 2.1).

The inner dermis layer contains blood vessels, lymph ducts, nerve fibers and nerve endings, hair follicles, and glands. The job of these glands is to produce sweat to keep you cool and to create an oily substance called *sebum* that helps prevent the skin from drying out. Sweat and sebum get to the skin's surface through tiny holes called *pores*.

The outer epidermis is thinner than the dermis and is made up of *squamous* cells (also known as keratinocytes). Beneath these squamous cells are fuller shaped cells called *basal* cells. Basal cells are constantly dividing and rise to the top of the epidermis

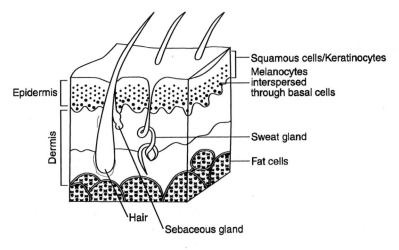

Figure 2.1 A cross-section of your skin

where they are programmed to die and become the dead outer layer of our skin, known as the *stratum corneum*. Underneath and interspersed between the basal cells are *melanocytes*.

Melanocytes produce *melanin*, a pigment that gives skin and hair its color. The more melanin in your skin, the darker it is. For example, people of African descent have more melanin in their skin than people of Norwegian descent. The importance of melanin is that it absorbs the ultraviolet radiation of the sun, thus protecting the skin cells against sunburn. Because dark-skinned people are "designed" to live in sunny regions, those with darker skin produce melanin all the time, whereas light-skinned people mainly produce melanin only in response to sun exposure. As you're about to find out, however, everyone who produces melanin in their skin—which is everyone except very fair-skinned or freckled, red-haired persons—has a natural defense against the sun's radiation.

How Your Skin Tans . . . and Burns

One of the most important jobs of the epidermis—especially for light-skinned people—is to adapt quickly to protect skin cells from the sun's radiation. The defense mechanism the skin uses against sunburn is what we call "tanning," which is an ingenious process. In response to sun exposure, the melanocytes produce melanin pigment that makes the skin darker. This protects the skin because melanin pigment absorbs UV radiation. Even short bursts of sun exposure will trigger the melanocytes to produce more melanin pigment.

Dark-skinned people do not have more melanocytes, but their melanocytes are more active, which explains why their skin is always pigmented. It also explains why the risk of all forms of skin cancer is lower for dark-skinned people—the cells of their skin are always more protected from sunburn by the presence of melanin pigment, which acts like an umbrella, shielding the cell's vulnerable DNA from UV damage due to sun exposure.

Sun*burn* is quite different from a sun*tan*. When you get a sunburn, your skin turns red and can sometimes blister and peel. This redness, known in scientific terms as *erythema*, is actually caused by increased blood flow to the skin. This begins approximately four hours after the sun exposure and reaches its peak between eight and twenty-four hours after exposure.

Blood is being sent to the skin to attend to cells that have been damaged by the sun. When severely damaged squamous and basal cells cannot repair themselves, they "commit suicide" so they won't replicate in a mutated state and cause cancer. This form of cell suicide is known as *apoptosis*, or programmed

Skin Cancer Facts and Fallacies

Many myths are associated with skin cancer thanks to the barrage of public misinformation on this topic.

The Fallacies

Any and all sun exposure causes skin cancer. UVB radiation from sunlight is thought to be one of the causes of non-melanoma skin cancer—especially chronic overexposure to sunlight. However, science doesn't fully understand what the connection is. Because humans can't live *without* UVB radiation, this statement needs to be questioned.

Sun exposure is the main cause of melanoma. There is no scientific evidence that regular, moderate sun exposure causes melanoma. As the FDA observed after a 1995 conference on melanoma, the relationship between melanoma and sunlight is baffling. Melanoma is seen more often in people who *do not* receive regular, moderate sun exposure than in those who spend time in the sun. Melanomas also usually occur on parts of the body that receive no sun exposure. This suggests that genetics plays a much more important role in the development of melanoma than does regular, moderate sun exposure. There is also evidence that UVB-protection-only sunscreens may distort the UVB/UVA ratio that penetrates into the skin, thus contributing to melanoma development.

We are in the midst of a skin cancer "epidemic." It is inaccurate to call the increasing incidence of skin cancer an epidemic. Skin cancer rates have been rising steadily since the early twentieth century.

Skin cancer rates are going up solely because more people are sunbathing. Although skin cancer rates have been rising steadily since the early twentieth century, it wasn't until the 1960s that a tanned skin was considered desirable. Present-day people actually spend *less* time outdoors than did our forebears, most of whom worked the land before the industrial revolution. Working outdoors throughout the year probably helped

(continues)

Skin Cancer Facts and Fallacies (*continued*)

previous generations build a resistance to sunburn in the form of tanned skin. More recently—especially in the 1970s and 1980s, when a severe sunburn was considered a prerequisite for an eventual summer tan—people have become more likely to get sunburned, which is thought to be one of the main causes of melanoma. In addition, the use of UVB-protection-only sunscreens probably contributed to the rise of melanoma because they promoted massive exposure to UVA.

There's no such thing as a safe tan. Tanned skin protects you against sunburn, thought to be the main cause of melanoma. Also, it's more dangerous to avoid sun exposure completely than it is to get regular, moderate sun exposure. If you avoid getting sunburned, the benefits of sun exposure will far outweigh the possible dangers. Independent scientific research has shown that if you live in a sunny climate, or if you live in a not-so-sunny climate but expose yourself to sun, then your increased production of vitamin D due to UVB radiation will help lower risk of a host of debilitating and fatal diseases.

Tanning is like smoking to your skin. Wrong. Tanning is natural. It is your body's natural defense against sunburn. Smoking is an unnatural habit that your body rejects by becoming ill.

The Facts

Sun exposure may actually prevent cancer. Numerous published studies show that regular, moderate sun exposure helps prevent several forms of cancer. Cancer rates in higher latitudes, where there is less sun exposure over the course of the year, are higher than in sunnier climes. Furthermore, both men and women who live in higher latitudes who make an effort to be exposed to more sunlight decrease their risk of getting these common, lethal cancers.

(continues)

Skin Cancer Facts and Fallacies *(continued)*

Cancerwise, the benefits of sun exposure outweigh the risks.
Non-melanoma skin cancer has an extremely low death rate. In the
United States, it claims about 1,200 lives a year. Colon, prostate, and
breast cancer—which together claim about 175,000 lives—can in some
cases be prevented by regular, moderate sun exposure. People who get
regular, moderate sun exposure are less likely to get a malignant
melanoma than those who don't.

It's a scientific fact: If you get regular, moderate sun exposure, you
have less chance of developing malignant melanoma. New research
shows that melanoma is more prevalent in Europe and North America
than in the equatorial latitudes, which again suggests that regular sun exposure may prevent melanoma. At the very least, moderate sun exposure
will not increase the risk of melanoma.

cell death. However, severely damaged melanocytes stay alive,
and these cells may replicate in a mutated way, resulting in the
formation of a melanoma later in life.

What Is Skin Cancer?

Our bodies function normally when the cells that make up the
different groups of tissue—such as the prostate, breast, and
colon—grow, divide, and replace themselves in an orderly fashion. Occasionally, cells divide too rapidly and multiply out of
control; this can lead to cancer. Skin cancer results when this
process occurs in the cells of the skin.

There are several forms of skin cancer, but all of them fit into two broad categories: non-melanoma skin cancer and melanoma.

Non-Melanoma Skin Cancer

By far the most common forms of non-melanoma skin cancer are *basal cell carcinoma* and *squamous cell carcinoma* ("carcinoma" is the medical term for cancer).

Basal Cell Carcinoma   Basal cell carcinoma (BCC) affects the basal cells in the epidermis and is the most common form of non-melanoma skin cancer. BCC usually occurs on areas of your skin that are most exposed to the sun and that have most likely been sunburned, such as the nose, face, tops of the ears, and backs of the hands. Often BCC appears as a small raised bump that has a smooth, "pearly" appearance. Sometimes BCC looks like a scar and feels firm when you press on it. BCC may expand in size and spread to tissues around it, but these cells rarely spread to other parts of the body.

Squamous Cell Carcinoma   Squamous cell carcinoma (SCC) also occurs on areas of the epidermis that are most often exposed to extreme amounts of sun. Often SCC appears as a firm red bump. Sometimes the tumor may feel dry, itchy, and scaly, may bleed, or may develop a crust. SCC very occasionally spreads to nearby lymph nodes (lymph nodes produce and store infection-fighting immune cells). SCC may also appear on parts of your skin that have been burned, exposed to chemicals, or had X-ray therapy or PUVA treatments for psoriasis (see chapter 4).

What Is Actinic Keratosis?

You may have heard of actinic keratosis. President George W. Bush was treated for actinic keratosis on his face in 2002. This skin condition is not cancer, but in some people it can change into basal cell or squamous cell carcinoma. Actinic keratosis occurs as rough white, red, or brown scaly patches on the skin, usually in areas that have been exposed to the sun. Treatment of actinic keratosis requires removal of the affected skin cells. New skin then forms from deeper healthy basal cells that have escaped sun damage. Treatment of actinic keratosis is usually successful if it is detected early on.

Melanoma

Melanoma is a different story. Although rare, melanoma is much more deadly than non-melanoma skin cancer. Comprising only 10 percent of all skin cancers, melanomas are responsible for 85 percent of skin cancer deaths, killing about 7,000 Americans annually.

Melanomas occur in the deeper pigment-producing cells located between the dermis and epidermis, known as the melanocytes. When melanocytes become cancerous, or *malignant*, these cells grow uncontrollably and aggressively invade surrounding healthy tissues. Melanoma may stay in the skin, but more often it spreads, or *metastasizes*, through the blood or lymph system to the bones and organs, including the brain, lungs, and liver.

Melanoma sometimes occurs in an existing mole or other skin blemish such as a dysplastic nevi (pronounced dis-PLAS-tik

NEE-vye), but it often develops in otherwise unmarked skin. In men, melanoma develops most often on the upper back, and in women it is usually seen on the legs, although it may occur anywhere. Melanoma is most common in people with fair skin and those who have a large number of moles, although it affects people of all races.

Melanoma usually resembles a flat, brown or black mole with an irregular, uneven border. Usually the blemish is not symmetrical. Melanoma lesions are often 6 millimeters (0.24 inches) or more in diameter. Any change in the shape, size, or color of a mole may indicate melanoma. A melanoma may be lumpy or rounded, change color, become crusty, ooze, or bleed.

Skin Type and Cancer Risk

Because melanin pigment protects skin cells against the damaging effects of the sun, certain people have higher rates of skin cancer than others. People with fairer skin (less-pigmented/less-protected) have a higher rate of skin cancer than people with darker skin (more-pigmented/more-protected).

Scientists have categorized skin into six different types based on melanin pigment content. Refer to page 39 to find out what skin type you are. People with Type 1 skin have the highest risk of skin cancer, and people with Type 6 skin, the lowest risk. If you have Type 1 or Type 2 skin and were exposed to excessive amounts of sun as a child, adolescent, or adult—including several severe sunburns—you are in the highest risk group for skin cancer and should get screened.

Some people never get tan, principally those who are very fair-skinned or red-haired and freckled. They have what's

What Skin Type Am I?

If you don't know your skin type and, thus, your relative risk for skin cancer, refer to the following table.

I always burn, never tan, and am fair with red or blond hair and freckles (albinos, some redheads).	I have **Type 1 skin.**
I easily burn, hardly get tan, and am fair skinned (people of northern European origin, such as Scandinavians or Celts).	I have **Type 2 skin.**
I occasionally burn and gradually tan (people of Mediterranean and Middle East origin).	I have **Type 3 skin.**
I rarely burn and always tan (people of East Asian origin and some Indians and Pakistanis).	I have **Type 4 skin.**
I seldom burn, always tan, and have medium-to-dark skin (people of African origin, South East Asians, and some Indians and Pakistanis).	I have **Type 5 skin.**
I never burn and tan darkly (people with "blue-black" skin, of African origin, and dark-skinned Asians such as Tamils).	I have **Type 6 skin.**

known as Type 1 skin. The reason people with Type 1 skin don't tan is because the melanocytes in their skin are unable to produce protective melanin pigment. Because their skin is unprotected against the sun's radiation, these people are highly susceptible to sun damage, including sunburn, and are therefore at the highest risk for skin cancer.

What Causes Skin Cancer?

Confusion exists about what causes skin cancer. The two main forms of skin cancer—non-melanoma skin cancer and melanoma—have different causes. But much of the information out there lumps these two very different forms of skin cancer together in such a way that it would erroneously appear that they have an identical cause—sun exposure. Because some sunshine is vital for the health and very survival of humans, it is important to sort out the confusion.

Causes of Non-Melanoma Skin Cancer

Non-melanoma skin cancer is thought to be caused by long-term exposure to sunshine. Such exposure over many years may cause damage to the skin cells themselves so they eventually start replicating out of control. Sun exposure over many years may also desensitize the skin's immune system in such a way that it will not recognize and act against cancerous skin cells. Finally, researchers have been looking at the p53 gene, a "quality control" gene system that is responsible for fixing a damaged cell or causing it to kill itself (apoptosis). There is mounting evidence that the p53 gene system may be damaged by excessive, long-term sun exposure. Each person has two p53 genes—one from each parent. When one p53 gene is damaged, the skin cell becomes sick and multiplies abnormally to form a precancerous scaly lesion known as an actinic keratosis (see page 37). When both p53 genes are damaged and can no longer function properly, the skin cell may start replicating out of control and become a non-melanoma skin cancer. The p53 gene is

What Is XP?

Xeroderma pigmentosum (XP) is an extremely rare skin disorder whose sufferers are highly sensitive to sun exposure. The cause of XP is hypersensitivity of the skin cells to UV radiation due to a defect in the gene's DNA repair system. People with XP experience premature aging of the skin and multiple skin cancers. The disease is usually diagnosed in infancy when the child with XP exhibits severe skin problems, including skin reddening, scaling, and freckling. Skin cancers usually appear in early childhood, as do chronic eye problems. There is no cure for this disease, and the only course of action is to stay out of the sun.

so important that it was declared the "Molecule of the Year" by the editors of the journal *Science* and is the only gene that has ever appeared on the cover of *Newsweek*!

The likelihood that you will develop non-melanoma skin cancer is greater if your exposure to sunshine began when you were a child, adolescent, or young adult. During these early years, the skin is especially vulnerable to the sun. Then there is also the simple fact that the earlier in life that skin cells are damaged, the longer the chance they have to replicate in a mutated state.

Remember, not everyone who is exposed to strong sunshine from a young age is going to develop non-melanoma skin cancer. Some people are genetically predisposed to this disease. This explains why certain people get non-melanoma skin cancer while others don't—even when they have the same skin type and are exposed to just about the same amount of sun. It's

---

Mechanism of Skin Cancer:
Non-Melanoma Skin Cancer Versus Melanoma

Non-melanoma skin cancer (rarely deadly, easily treated when caught early) is probably caused by long-term sun exposure starting early in life that damages squamous and basal skin cells and the p53 gene, which exists to prevent cells from replicating in a mutated form to cause cancerous growths

Melanoma skin cancer (often deadly, often treatable if caught early) is probably caused by (1) intermittent sunburns starting early in life that cause damage to the melanocytes; (2) multiple exposures to sunlight while wearing a UVB-only sunscreen, resulting in extreme exposure to UVA radiation; and (3) genetics, especially for those with a large number of moles (nevi).

---

also believed that a fatty diet may predispose you to a variety of cancers, including non-melanoma skin cancer.

Causes of Melanoma

There are numerous risk factors for melanoma. Radiation from the sun is but one. This explains why melanomas occur in people who don't spend time in the sun and why melanomas are often seen on parts of the body that often aren't exposed to the sun (see figure 2.2). Here are some of the nonradiation risk factors:

- **Heredity.** If two or more of your family members have had a melanoma, you are much more likely to get one.

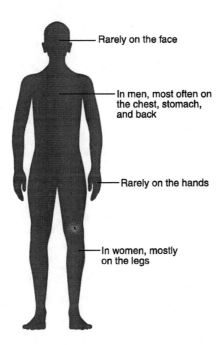

Rarely on the face

In men, most often on
the chest, stomach,
and back

Rarely on the hands

In women, mostly
on the legs

Figure 2.2 *Where do melanomas occur?* The fact that melanomas
tend to occur on areas of the body that are not as exposed to the
sun as others suggests that sun exposure is but one risk factor for
this disease. If sun exposure were the main cause of melanomas,
they would be seen mostly on the hands, face, ears, nose, etc.

- **Dysplastic nevi.** These kinds of moles are more likely
  than normal moles to become melanomas (see page 45).

- **Many normal moles.** If you have more than fifty moles
  on your body, this will increase your chance of developing a melanoma because melanoma usually begins in the
  melanocytes of a normal mole.

- **Weakened immune system.** People whose immune system is weakened by some other forms of cancer, certain

drugs such as cyclosporine prescribed after organ transplants, or AIDS have a greater risk of developing melanoma.

- **Previous melanoma.** People who have already had a melanoma are at a high risk for developing another.

- **Defective DNA repair system in XP.** Patients with XP (see page 41) tend to have a defective DNA repair system and are at a higher risk of melanoma.

This brings us to the relationship between sun exposure and melanoma. Normal sun exposure of the type that builds a tan doesn't seem to be responsible for melanoma. Numerous studies pioneered by Doctors Cedric and Frank Garland show that people who work outside have lower incidences of melanoma than do people who work inside. In one of these studies, the Garland brothers and their colleagues showed that Navy personnel who worked *above decks* on aircraft carriers were less likely to get melanomas than those who worked *below decks.* Despite the fact that the United States was for several centuries a rural, agricultural-based nation whose citizens were outdoors much of the time, melanoma was so rare that separate statistics weren't kept on the disease until the 1950s.

So what's going on? How come melanoma rates are increasing rapidly and have been doing so at a rate of 2 percent per year for more than thirty years?

The answer is surprising—it may be because people are exposed to sunshine *less* during their working hours. Sunburns are a risk factor for melanoma. Because people these days—young and old alike—work outside less and therefore get less regular sun exposure than did previous generations, they are at in-

Moles and Dysplastic Nevi

Clusters of melanocytes and surrounding tissue sometimes join to form a noncancerous growth called a mole (in medical terms, a *nevus*, the plural of which is *nevi*). Most of us have between ten and forty moles, which can be flesh-colored, pink, tan, or brown. Moles can be flat or raised. Usually symmetrical, moles are round or oval and smaller than a pencil eraser. Moles may be present at birth or may appear later in life—usually before age forty. In general, moles change very little, although they tend to fade away as you get older. When moles are surgically removed, they usually do not return.

Some moles look very different from common moles. *Dysplastic nevi* are generally larger than ordinary moles and have irregular and indistinct borders. Their color is often mottled, ranging from pink to dark brown. Usually dysplastic nevi are flat, but areas may be raised above the skin surface.

A person who has a lot of moles (more than fifty) or who has dysplastic nevi is at increased risk of developing melanoma.

creased risk of getting sunburned rather than suntanned when they *do* go out in the sun.

Another explanation for the rise of melanoma may surprise you even more: the use of sunscreens starting in the 1950s.

Before any of you heave your sunscreens into the trash, let me make the point that the type of sunscreen that probably contributed to the rise of melanoma is the kind that protected only against UVB radiation. Until the late 1990s, UVB-protection-only sunscreen was all that was available, and this had been the case since the 1940s. In the past few years, this type of sunscreen has been phased out in favor of sunscreens that protect against UVB *and* UVA radiation.

Sunscreen was first developed to enable people to avoid sunburn and thereby spend more time in the sun either tanning or participating in outdoor recreation. Although these early sunscreens protected against the burning radiation of UVB, they did not protect against UVA radiation. At the time, UVA radiation was not thought to be harmful because it didn't cause the obvious symptoms of sunburn. The increase in melanoma may partially be due to the fact that by protecting people against UVB, UVB-only sunscreen use enables people to receive massive doses of UVA, which penetrates deep into the epidermis and dermis to damage the melanocytes.

We now know that UVA is partially responsible for melanoma, and the cosme-ceutical industry has introduced sunscreens that protect against both UVB *and* UVA radiation— so-called broad-spectrum sunscreens. You should always use broad-spectrum sunscreens when trying to prevent sunburn.

With all this in mind, it is important to remember that melanoma usually occurs in parts of the body that are not exposed to the sun and is seen in people who do not spend much time in the sun, two factors that indicate that sun exposure may not be a risk factor for this serious disease.

Skin Cancer Detection

Almost all forms of skin cancer are easily treated with favorable outcomes *if they are caught early on.* Even the rare but potentially fatal melanoma form of skin cancer can be managed successfully and even cured if it is detected in its early stages.

The key to early detection and treatment of skin cancer is very much in your hands. There's no need for panic or overreaction, but you need to be on the lookout and know what to look for.

The same way women should do a regular breast self-exam, each person should periodically check his or her skin for possible early signs of skin cancer. How often you do this depends on your risk factors. If you or a close relative has a history of skin cancer, or if other risk factors apply to you—such as if you have Type 1 or Type 2 skin and had a lot of sun exposure as a child—examine your skin once a month. Otherwise, once every six months is probably sufficient. Checking yourself every day is counterproductive because you may not notice subtle changes that could be signs of skin cancer. Specific guidelines on how to do a skin self-exam are on page 49.

What to Look For

A red flag for skin cancer is a change in your skin's appearance, such as a new growth or a sore that doesn't heal.

Look for these warning signs that you might have a non-melanoma skin cancer:

- A lump that is small, smooth, shiny, and "waxy" looking

- A lump that is firm and red

- A lump that bleeds or develops a crusty surface

- A flat, red area that is rough, dry, itchy, or scaly

- A scar-like growth that gradually gets larger

The Warning Signs of Melanoma Skin Cancer

An effective way to remember the warning signs of a melanoma is to use this ABCD checklist:

A—Asymmetry: one half is unlike the other half

B—Border irregular: scalloped or poorly circumscribed border

C—Color varied from one area to another: shades of tan and brown; black; sometimes white, red, or blue

D—Diameter: larger than the diameter of a pencil eraser (6 mm)

If you see any of these changes on your skin, consult your personal physician immediately to determine their cause.

What about signs for melanoma? This very rare but dangerous form of skin cancer generally begins as an irregular-shaped, flat blemish colored a mottled light brown to black. Melanomas are usually at least one-quarter inch across. The blemish may crust on the surface and bleed. Melanomas usually appear on the upper back, torso, bellybutton, back of the legs, lower legs, head, or neck. Seek medical attention for a mole that changes size, shape, or color; a new mole; or a mole that looks odd or unpleasant or begins to grow.

Remember that pain is not an indicator of a skin cancer. Until it progresses to quite an advanced stage, a skin cancer won't hurt or sting. This fact reinforces the need to see a doctor as soon as you have any legitimate suspicion.

How to Look for Skin Cancer

A good time to do a self-exam is after a shower or bath. Examine yourself in a well-lit room using a full-length and a hand-held mirror. If you don't own a full-length mirror, use a three-way mirror in a private, well-lit dressing room at a clothing store. Start by learning where your birthmarks, moles, and blemishes are and what they look like. Check for anything new—a change in the size, texture, or color of a mole, or a sore that won't heal.

The following are some other tips:

- Check everywhere, including your back, bellybutton, between your buttocks, and your genitals (remember—melanomas often occur in non-sun-exposed parts of your body).

- Examine the front and back of your body in the mirror, then raise your arms and look at the left and right sides.

- Bend your elbows and look carefully at your palms, the top and underside of your hands and forearms, and your upper arms.

- Look at the front and back of your legs.

- Sit and closely inspect your feet, including between your toes.

- Examine your face, neck, and scalp. If necessary, use a comb or blow dryer to move your hair so you can see better.

What If You Find Something?

If you examine your skin regularly, you will become familiar with what on your body is normal. If you find anything suspicious (refer to page 47) during the course of your examination, see your doctor right away. Remember, the earlier skin cancer is found, the more straightforward the treatment program is and the greater the chance for successful resolution.

If a doctor thinks a growth looks suspicious, he or she will order a "biopsy." In this simple office procedure, the patient is given a local anesthetic, and all or some of the suspect tissue is removed and examined under a microscope.

If skin cancer is diagnosed, there are various options for treatment. The doctor's goal will be to totally remove or destroy the cancer while leaving as small a scar as possible. Types of surgery include cryosurgery (destruction by freezing with liquid nitrogen), laser surgery (using a laser beam to cut away or vaporize growths), and curettage and electrodesiccation (using a spoonlike blade to scoop out the growth, followed by destruction of surrounding tissue with an electric needle). Occasionally other treatments, such as radiation therapy or chemotherapy, may be used alone or in combination.

Precise treatment and follow-up for both non-melanoma skin cancer and melanoma depends on a variety of factors, including the cancer's location and size; the risk of scarring; and the person's age, health, and medical history. All of this is too complex to comprehensively cover in this book. An excellent resource for information on skin cancer treatment is the National Cancer Institute. You can access their Web site at www.cancer.gov/CancerInformation/CancerType/skin.

Again, the most important thing to know about treatment is that the earlier you catch skin cancer, the more straightforward and successful the treatment will be.

Preventing Skin Cancer

One of the characteristics of skin cancer is that, unlike all other cancers, it is *visible*. If everyone were vigilant about detecting skin cancer in its early stages through self-exams, the mortality rate for this disease—especially non-melanoma skin cancer—would go down to virtually zero.

We know how to catch skin cancer in its early stages, which is the key to reducing its severity. What can we do to prevent skin cancer from occurring at all?

Non-Melanoma Skin Cancer Prevention

The regrettable fact is that almost all the damage from the sun occurs in childhood and early adulthood. If you're older than thirty, most of the sun damage that might have contributed to your risk of non-melanoma skin cancer and melanoma has already taken place. Still, you can reduce your risk of skin cancer to some extent by being judicious about how much sun exposure you get in the future. Although sun exposure and sunburn early in life don't mean you will necessarily get skin cancer, your chances are higher. Therefore, from the age of thirty onward you should focus on early detection. It's also important to educate younger family members about the risks of skin damage from long-term sun exposure and intermittent sunburn. Explain to them how they can safely get the benefits of sun exposure (see chapter 7).

Folks over age seventy need not worry about trying to prevent skin cancer by staying out of the sun. In people of this age who have spent a lot of time in the sun, the damage has almost certainly been done. In addition to vigilance in regard to skin cancer detection, the concern among older people should be whether they are getting *enough* sun to achieve and maintain healthy vitamin D levels (see chapter 1). Older people are much more likely to die from a vitamin D deficiency–related hip fracture due to osteoporosis than from skin cancer.

If you *are* younger than thirty and have had a great deal of unprotected sun exposure in your life, you should avoid any more UV exposure than is necessary to maintain good health (chapter 7 provides specific guidelines on how much unprotected sunshine you need). It is especially important that you protect against sunburn.

Preventing Excess Sun Exposure and Sunburn

You can prevent excess sun exposure and sunburn by applying a high-SPF broad-spectrum sunscreen (15 or more) *after* getting the minimum amount of sun exposure you need to build and maintain vitamin D levels (remember that SPF8 and SPF15 sunscreens reduce vitamin D production by 97.5 percent and 99.9 percent, respectively). Follow the directions on the sunscreen label to make sure you use the correct amount. SPF refers to the length of time a particular product protects against skin reddening from UVB exposure compared to skin without protection. For example, if your skin takes twenty minutes to begin reddening without protection, applying an SPF15 sun-

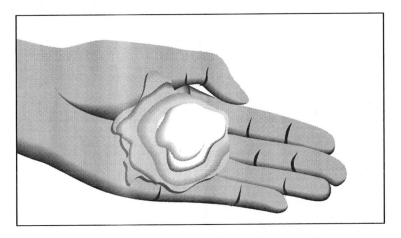

Figure 2.3 One ounce, or a large handful, of sunscreen is what a typical swimsuit-clad adult needs to get the SPF protection stated on the label.

screen should prevent reddening fifteen times longer—about five hours (though it may take up to twenty-four hours after sun exposure for redness to become visible). To maintain the SPF protection, it is important to reapply sunscreen every four hours and always after swimming.

To get the SPF advertised on the product label, an adult in a bathing suit typically needs to use fully *one-quarter* of a four-ounce bottle of sunscreen to cover his or her body (see figure 2.3). Studies have consistently shown that people do not apply enough sunscreen, which means they are not getting the protection they think they are.

Special care should be taken if you have Type 1 skin, if you haven't been exposed to the sun for some time, if you go out during peak summer months, or if you live at high altitude (especially if there is snow on the ground, which reflects UV radiation).

In addition to wearing sunscreen, you can also take the following measures:

- Wear tight-woven clothing. Long sleeves, long trousers, or a long skirt should be worn. Tests have shown such clothing blocks UV radiation much more effectively than do sunscreens.

- Wear a broad-brimmed hat.

- Try to stay in the shade.

Melanoma Prevention

Severe sunburn before the age of thirty is one of the risk factors for melanoma later in life. Protecting your children against sunburn needs to be a priority in your household. In addition, be especially vigilant about sun exposure if you haven't been exposed to strong sunshine for some time. This typically happens to people in northern states in the springtime or summer when their skin has little protective pigment in it after the long winter. However, it can happen to a person anytime and anywhere if he or she hasn't been out in the sun for an extended period and then goes out in the strong sunshine—whether it's to sail, play tennis, or work in the garden or on the roof. Sunburn is also common in people from northern climates who take their winter break vacations in sunny, warm places such as the Caribbean.

People with Type 1 and Type 2 skin need to be especially vigilant because they are at much greater risk of getting sunburned and, therefore, at much greater risk of developing melanoma.

Improve Your Diet and Prevent Skin Cancer

Eating a healthy diet is a little-known but extremely important way to prevent skin cancer. A 1995 study published in the *International Journal of Cancer* reported that people who ate a low-fat diet had 90 percent less chance of getting skin cancer. Conversely, a diet high in fat shortens the time between UV exposure and the onset of cancer and increases the number of tumors that develop. According to this same article, the magnitude of the dietary effect is almost directly related to the amount and kind of fat consumed (saturated fat appears to be related to skin cancer).

Unfortunately, for a century now, the American diet has been getting higher in fat—especially in the extra-unhealthy saturated fats. This may partly explain why skin cancer rates have gone up. The average American diet is about 16 percent saturated fat, whereas most qualified dieticians will tell you it should be no more than one-third of that. To make matters worse, there has been a trend toward fad weight-loss programs advocating high fat content (the Atkins Diet is probably the best known of these). Leaving aside whether these diets actually work in the long term to help people keep weight off, diets high in saturated fat may cause a variety of life-threatening health problems and probably contribute to skin cancer.

To reduce your risk of skin cancer, you should start eating a diet that is low in fat, especially saturated fat. There are several excellent eating plans out there that advocate eating this way. One of the best of these is the DASH diet, based on the highly successful government-sponsored study called Dietary Approaches to Stop Hypertension, which was spearheaded by a Boston University Medical Center colleague of mine, Dr. Tom Moore.

Let's Hear It for the Human Body

We need to give the human body more credit than it sometimes gets. People don't shrivel, shatter, or shut down at the first sign of stress. Instead, the human body operates on the "overload principle"—when subjected to outside forces, it adapts by getting stronger. Let's use the exercise analogy again. Your muscles don't pop and your bones don't break if you regularly lift weights—they get bigger and more powerful. Your heart and lungs don't explode or collapse if you go running every morning—they become more efficient. Your ligaments and tendons don't snap if you do stretching exercises—they get more flexible.

The same goes with your skin's exposure to sunshine. If your skin receives regular, moderate exposure to sunshine, it adapts by producing melanin to absorb the sun's radiation, thereby protecting itself against a future burn. This is the human body's natural adaptation to outside stress. Of course, sudden and extreme exposure to strong sunshine after an extended period of nonexposure will result in sunburn in the same way that exposure to sudden and extreme physical activity can result in damage to the muscle-bone system or the heart.

Remember, too, that skin did not evolve solely to resist the power of the sunshine—your skin is the very conduit through which your body uses the sun's radiation to create the vitamin D you need for your very survival.

Plus you have an entire DNA repair system made up of enzymes whose job is to repair damaged DNA and replace it with healthy new material. My colleagues and I are doing research to determine if the skin's DNA repair program is enhanced when it is exposed to moderate sunlight, and I suspect that it does.

All this is to say that your body is designed to accommodate the effects of sunshine. To suggest that sunshine is necessarily harmful to your skin is to underestimate the human species' ability to adapt to its environment.

Unconfusing the Issue

Anti-sun activists argue that to differentiate between the causes of non-melanoma skin cancer and melanoma is to confuse the issue—they maintain that you need to avoid all sunshine and become a sun-phobe. This ignores the fact that some sun exposure is necessary to *survive* and be *healthy*. The amount of sun exposure that causes the potentially deadly melanoma—sunburn—should be stringently avoided, but the moderate, regular sun exposure, which is your main source of vitamin D and which is associated with the rarely deadly and easily treated non-melanoma skin cancer, should not be forsaken. If it is, you increase your risk of developing a variety of more serious and deadly diseases.

Some people enjoy being in the sun and using indoor tanning facilities so much that they will risk non-melanoma skin cancer in favor of all the potential benefits of sun exposure. Others may choose to get only the minimum amount of UVB exposure necessary to build and maintain vitamin D levels (you can find specific guidelines for this in chapter 7). These are choices only you can make. However, we know a couple of things for sure. Subjecting yourself to unlimited amounts of UVB is potentially harmful. But denying yourself any and all UVB can lead to serious health problems.

CHAPTER THREE

Sunlight and
Skin Appearance

*How to avoid wrinkles and
other skin problems and still
get the health benefits of sunshine*

WHETHER I AM at a cocktail party or a baseball game, when people find out I am a professor of dermatology, they inevitably ask: "What do I do about my wrinkles?" In our youth-obsessed culture, some people will go to extraordinary lengths to eliminate the creases and crinkles on their faces. Cosmetic surgery, chemical peels, and injections of Botox or collagen are but a few of the drastic measures folks take to treat wrinkles.

Preventing wrinkles is another fixation. You only have to peruse the shelves of any pharmacy to see the volume of lotions and potions being sold that supposedly prevent wrinkles. The most frequent course of action taken by many people who wish to avoid getting wrinkles is to shun exposure to sunlight. True sun-phobes behave as if even momentary exposure to sunlight will transform them into shriveled prunes—they refuse to go outside without covering themselves in sun protection creams, hats, wraparound sunglasses, and long sleeves and pants to walk to the corner store for a gallon of milk.

It is true that *excessive* sun exposure is one of the reasons people develop wrinkles earlier and eventually become more wrinkled than they would otherwise, a process known as "photoaging." Concern about skin appearance is harmless, but when this pursuit is taken to an extreme by depriving oneself of sun, there can be harmful consequences. Along with exaggerated concerns about skin cancer, concern about getting wrinkles from the sun is a major cause of the epidemic of vitamin D deficiency in the United States and the Western world.

As you'll find out in this chapter, the good news is, you can get the health benefits of sun exposure and at the same time minimize the cosmetic harm to your skin. First let's look at the reasons people get wrinkles.

What Causes Wrinkles?

Wrinkles are a natural part of aging. Every single one of us will get wrinkles. There are a variety of reasons why we develop wrinkles as we get older. Your skin, which is constantly regenerating and repairing itself throughout your life, becomes less efficient at doing so the older you get. The inner skin, your dermis, gets thinner. Also, the underlying layer of elastin and collagen fibers, which gives young skin its springiness, starts to break down. Your skin's moisture retention capabilities also diminish, causing it to become dry and scaly.

How wrinkled you get depends on a combination of genetic, environmental, and lifestyle factors.

Detecting Sun Damage Using a UV Camera

Visual evidence of how much sun damage your skin has undergone can be gained using a UV camera (refer to page 72). This device functions rather like a black-and-white Polaroid camera. The light penetrates 1 mm below the skin surface, exposing the damage in the form of black dots, which is where the melanin has clumped. *This process does not detect cancer.* For comparison, another picture is also taken using a regular lens on the camera.

Genetics

Many of the changes in the collagen and elastin that give your skin its firmness and elasticity depend on genetic factors you can do nothing about—they are inherited from your parents who inherited them from *their* parents. Because each person has a different genetic program, loss of skin firmness and elasticity takes place differently from person to person.

The Environment

The most important environmental cause of premature wrinkles is excessive exposure to the sun's UVA radiation. Wind and pollution can damage the skin too, especially if your exposure to these elements is extreme. Ironically, as with melanoma, the wrinkled skin you see in many baby boomers may be a result of the advent of sunscreens in the 1960s. Why? These early sunscreens protected people from UVB radiation—which causes burning—enabling them to spend lengthy periods in the sun.

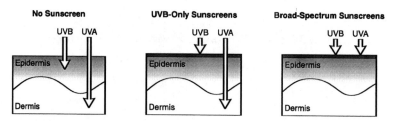

Figure 3.1 Old-fashioned UVB-only sunscreens block UVB radiation that is thought to cause non-melanoma skin cancer, but they let in UVA radiation that has been linked to melanoma. Newer broad-spectrum sunscreens block both UVB *and* UVA radiation and are the products recommended when you will be in the sun longer than the time recommended for making vitamin D.

However, these UVB-protection-only products did nothing to protect against UVA radiation because at the time UVA radiation wasn't thought to have any effect. We now know, however, that it is mostly the UVA radiation from sunshine that causes the damage responsible for wrinkles (see figure 3.1). Thus, early sunscreens contributed to premature wrinkling in people who used them because they enabled these people to spend long periods in the sun without getting burned. In doing so, these folks were exposed to unnaturally large doses of UVA radiation.

Lifestyle

Most of us know that smoking causes lung cancer, heart disease, and stroke. What's not as well known is that smoking is also responsible for prematurely aged skin, the main characteristic of which is wrinkles. A study published in the *British Journal of Dermatology* in late 2002 showed that smoking has a more severe effect on the skin than does sun exposure.

Smoking causes wrinkles by interfering with the body's mechanism for breaking down old skin and renewing it. As a result, a forty-year-old person who smokes a pack of cigarettes a day has skin that makes the person look closer to sixty. The following are the telltale signs of aging caused by smoking:

- Lines or wrinkles spreading from the upper or lower lips or at right angles from the corners of the eyes (crow's-feet)

- Deep lines or numerous shallow lines on the cheeks and lower jaw

- Slight hollowness of the cheeks emphasizing the bony contours of the face and causing a gaunt appearance

- A leathery or worn appearance to the face, which may also have a grayish tinge

If you are concerned about your skin's appearance, then this is another reason not to smoke!

How to Minimize Wrinkles

Sunshine provides humans with essential vitamin D, which we need to survive. Yet we also now know that in extreme doses, the UVA radiation in sunlight can contribute to premature wrinkling. How can we balance the life-giving health benefits of sunlight with the desire to prevent wrinkles?

The most effective way to protect yourself against premature skin aging is to avoid excessive sun exposure—especially if you know you are predisposed to wrinkles because your parents

Minimize Face Wrinkles and Still Make Enough Vitamin D

My studies have shown that you can get your daily vitamin D requirement by exposing your face, hands, and arms (or arms and legs) to the sunlight for 25 to 50 percent of "1MED" (the time it takes you to get "pink" from the sun). See chapter 7 for a complete description and guidelines for finding your own optimal exposure time. I selected those particular areas of the body because they are the most convenient for gaining exposure to sunshine during normal daily activities. If you want to minimize the amount of wrinkling to your face—the area people are most sensitive about—expose a comparable area of skin in another part of your body such as your legs, stomach, or back.

became prematurely wrinkled. Remember, UVB-protection-only sunscreen will actually *increase* the damage to the cells responsible for your skin's elasticity, so it's important to use broad-spectrum sunscreens that protect against both UVA and UVB exposure.

What is "excessive exposure"? Anything more than the minimum amount you need to establish and maintain vitamin D levels could be considered excessive. Chapter 7 provides specific guidelines on how much unprotected sun exposure you need for good health, depending on your skin type, geographical location, and the time of year. Some people love the way sun and indoor tanning equipment make them feel. These people are willing to put up with wrinkles and other signs of photoaging, and they accept the increased risk of non-melanoma skin cancer associated with long-term UVB exposure (remember, non-melanoma skin cancer is very rarely fatal). This choice isn't totally unreasonable. If you make this decision, however, then definitely avoid sunburn, which is thought to be one of the main causes of deadly melanoma.

Other Indications of Aging Skin

For most people, wrinkles are the most obvious and worrisome sign of aging skin. However, other signs of aging manifest themselves in the skin as well, and, like wrinkles, they tend to be a combination of genetics and environment. Let's take a closer look at a few of the most common signs of aging skin.

"Liver" Spots (Lentigines)

Sometimes known as "age spots," these flat, brown patches with rounded edges tend to occur on the skin of the face, hands, back, and feet. They are a natural consequence of aging but may be exacerbated by sun exposure. They have nothing to do with the liver and are called liver spots only because they are brown. Many people consider liver spots unattractive, but they are not a health hazard. Always keep in mind that any large, flat, dark area with irregular borders should be examined by a doctor to rule out melanoma. Liver spots can be made to fade by restricting sun exposure to the affected areas and regularly applying creams that mildly bleach or exfoliate the skin. These products include alpha hydroxy acids, vitamin C, retinoids, azelaic acid, and quinones. More effective treatments include chemical peels or laser therapy.

Actinic Keratoses

These rough, white, red, or brown scaly patches on the skin tend to be found on areas of the skin that are most exposed to the sun. They are especially common in the elderly and people with light complexions. Approximately 10 percent of actinic keratoses develop into squamous cell carcinoma. These growths may be removed by a dermatologist using cryotherapy (freezing with liquid nitrogen), electrical cautery (burning), or surgery. Growths may also be treated with topical medications such as retinoids, which stimulate skin regeneration.

Seborrheic Keratoses

These wartlike growths, which appear to be pasted to the skin's surface, come in a variety of colors—yellow, brown, black, or other colors. To the untrained eye, they may look like a melanoma. They are not cancerous or precancerous, and they can easily be removed if considered unsightly. The growths are generally removed surgically or by cryotherapy. Removal is straightforward and usually does not leave a scar. However, growths on the trunk can leave lighter-colored skin. Seborrheic keratoses usually do not recur after removal, but people who are susceptible to them may develop others in the future.

Cherry Hemangiomas

These harmless, pinhead-sized, cherry-red domes are caused by a collection of dilated blood vessels. They develop in almost 90 percent of middle-aged to elderly people, usually on the torso. A dermatologist can remove them by surgery, cryotherapy, electrosurgery/cautery, or laser. Removal usually does not cause scarring.

Telangiectasias (Spider Veins)

Fine, reddish-blue veins on your nose, chin, or cheeks are a normal part of aging, but they may also be caused by sun damage, liver disease, pregnancy, birth control pills, estrogen replacement therapy, and even corticosteroids. They can be treated by a dermatologist with a laser.

Bruising

As you get older, your skin loses its fat padding, the blood vessels lose some of their resilience, and the skin becomes more vulnerable to damage. This usually manifests itself in bruising, which is actually bleeding under the skin. Bruising may be exacerbated by certain drugs, including aspirin, nonsteroidal anti-inflammatories (NSAIDs) such as Motrin, and the blood-thinning medications Coumadin and Plavix. Bruises that don't go away should be examined by your doctor.

Other Skin Diseases

Certain other skin diseases are more common in older people and are not related to sun exposure. These include shingles and leg ulcers due to poor circulation caused by diabetes or atherosclerosis.

Choosing a Dermatologist

If you decide you need to see a dermatologist for any reason, make sure he or she is board-certified in dermatology and has received continuing education in his or her specialty.

If you need a specific procedure performed, find out how many of those procedures the physician has performed. Request before-and-after photos of patients who have had the procedure.

The American Academy of Dermatology recommends you also look into the following issues:

- What outcome can be expected from the procedure?
- How long is the recuperation period?
- What are the risks and side effects of the procedure?
- Where is the procedure performed—office, outpatient facility, or hospital?
- What is the cost of the procedure? How will payment be required?

You should also find out if your health insurance will pay some or all of the cost.

Treating Cosmetic Skin Conditions

Sun-induced skin damage can be repaired or minimized in a number of ways. Repair options can be divided into three broad categories: implantations, resurfacing, and surgery. Let's look at each type of procedure and when it is most useful.

Implantations

Implantations can be used to treat crow's-feet and "whistle lines" around the lips. This kind of procedure is also effective in treating some scars. A number of different substances may be used, depending on your particular circumstance. Here are a few of the most common ones:

- **Collagen.** This is a natural bovine collagen extract. Patients need to be tested beforehand to rule out a possible allergy to this material. The substance is injected into the skin to plump up the area and thus reduce the appearance of a wrinkle. It is not a permanent solution, as the body gradually absorbs the foreign collagen and the wrinkle comes back.

- **Hyaluronic acid.** This is a collagen-derived substance used for lip augmentation and to reduce deeper furrows.

- **Fat injections.** Fat is extracted from the patient's own excess fat and is injected into the face to "plump" up the skin.

Resurfacing

Resurfacing can be used to treat fine lines, dryness, and blotchiness on the whole face. Again, several different substances are commonly used:

- **Alpha hydroxy acid.** A mild skin peel, this substance is often applied at night to stimulate skin regeneration.

- **Kinerase (furfurinyl acid).** This is a new antiaging preparation applied twice daily.

- **Topical retinoic acid (vitamin A).** Commonly found in cosmetic products such as "night cream," these items also help reverse photoaging and stimulate skin regeneration.

- **Glycolic acid peels.** This technique uses a series of superficial skin peels (sometimes known as "lunchtime peels" because they can be done so quickly and with minimum discomfort).

- **TCA peel.** This is a medium-depth peel that necessitates a week's home rest.

- **Erbium-YAG laser.** This is a medium-depth resurfacing process that necessitates a few days off from work for recovery.

- **Dermabrasion.** This technique works to smooth the skin using an electrical "sanding" machine.

- **C0$_2$/Erbium-YAG laser resurfacing.** Some of the most dramatic improvements have been seen using this new process, which removes the superficial layers of the skin layer by layer.

- **Nonablative resurfacing.** This is another promising new technology. A laser or radio device is used to burn or tighten the collagen without removing the surface skin—the skin texture improves with repeated treatment, but there is no "downtime."

Surgery

Surgery can be used to treat sagging and loose skin. Although this technique is perhaps best known because of celebrities' use of it, it is more costly and, as with any invasive procedure, involves greater risks. Anyone who decides to follow this course needs to proceed cautiously.

- A full face lift involves muscle/facial tightening for the jowls.

- A neck lift is performed to tighten the loose skin and muscles of the neck.

- A temporal (endoscopic) forehead lift is done to reduce sagging of the forehead and eyebrows.

- A blepharoplasty is performed to remove saggy eyelids.

Dr. Holick's New Treatment for Wrinkles

I have been working on a new therapy for wrinkles that is completely unlike anything currently available on the market.

In 1987, I found that a certain substance made by the skin cells inhibits excessive cell growth. This substance is called *parathyroid hormone-related peptide,* or PTHrP, and it exists in several forms. I tested a variety of PTHrPs in the hope of finding one—a so-called antagonist—that would reverse or block PTHrP's natural job of restricting cell growth. Eventually I did—it was PTH(7-34). It took a long time to develop this product because peptides are chemicals that are difficult to get into the skin. However, when we eventually developed a PTH(7-34) cream, it increased the skin plumpness of animals by an incredible 250 percent!

In human subjects, we anticipate that PTH(7-34) will make older skin less wrinkled, plumper, and more youthful-looking. In addition to cosmetic applications, we expect to be able to use PTH(7-34) to treat slow-healing wounds, which are common in older people.

We are about to start testing of PTH(7-34) in humans, and if the trials are successful, an effective antiwrinkle treatment product based on this substance will be on the market in three to four years.

(continues)

Dr. Holick's New Treatment for Wrinkles *(continued)*

I have also been evaluating a new vitamin infusion cream, known as MDT5, from the Somme Institute in New York City (www.sommeinstitute .com) that has been effective in reversing some of the sun damage in young women's faces. Figures 3.2 and 3.3 show before-and-after photos of a woman who used MDT5 over an eight-month period. The photos on the left are standard black-and-white photos; the photos on the right show UV images taken at the same time (see "Detecting Sun Damage Using a UV Camera" on page 61).

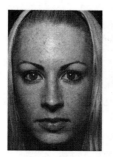 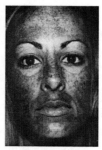

Figure 3.2 Pre-MDT5 treatment

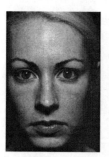 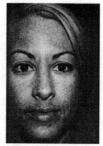

Figure 3.3 Post-MDT5 treatment

Looking Older and Feeling Good About It

Our culture is obsessed with youth, so it's hardly surprising that many of us are concerned about looking old. We can take certain steps to slow down the photoaging process, and many of these steps can increase our overall health as well. For those who wish to reverse the course of nature or take steps to remedy the consequences of a sun-drenched youth, some exciting new technologies are making this easier and less expensive. However, we all need to accept our physical appearance more than perhaps we do.

A thorough discussion of this high-minded notion is beyond the scope of this book. Suffice it to say that the best way to look and feel younger is to appreciate yourself for who you are and to have a positive outlook on life. By accepting themselves, people are doing more to make themselves attractive than all the cosmetic surgical procedures could!

CHAPTER FOUR

Sunshine Is Powerful Medicine

The good news about the healing power of the sun

CAN YOU IMAGINE what would happen if one of the drug companies came out with a single pill that reduced the risk of cancer, heart attack, stroke, osteoporosis, PMS, seasonal affective disorder, and various autoimmune disorders? There would be a media frenzy the likes of which has never been seen in response to a medical breakthrough! From the most sober newspapers would blare headlines like *"Miracle Pill" Will Save Millions of Lives* and *"Wonder Drug" Heralds New Age in Medicine.* The afternoon soap operas would be canceled so the networks could bring us continuing coverage of this discovery, and correspondents would be dispatched hither and yon to deliver breathless reportage.

Well, guess what? Such a drug exists, but it's not in pill form. If it's daytime, you can look out the window and see it in the sky. The "drug" I'm referring to, of course, is the sun.

Human beings have instinctively understood the relationship between sunshine and good health for thousands of years. In a famous hieroglyphic drawn during the time of the Egyptian pharaoh Akhenaten and his wife Nefertiti, the famed couple and their children were pictured being blessed by the many "hands" of the sun. The first few decades of the twentieth century were the heyday of photobiology and heliotherapy. Hospitals throughout Europe and North America built solariums so they could offer their patients a comfortable place to enjoy the sun's healing radiation for treating rickets, tuberculosis, and psoriasis. For demonstrating the health benefits of sunlight, photobiologist Dr. Niels Ryberg Finsen won the Nobel Prize for Medicine in 1903.

However, with the revelation that sunlight also contributed to skin cancer and prematurely aged skin, attitudes changed. Big money interests got behind the campaign to convince us that all sun is unhealthy so that people would always wear sunscreens and regularly visit the dermatologist. Thanks to the barrage of information that continues to be unleashed upon us, we became persuaded of this "fact."

It seems that the tide is about to change again. But don't slather yourself in baby oil and go running out to spend all day in the hot summer sun with a sun reflector. I encourage you to have a healthy respect for the consequences of overindulging. But you can begin once again to appreciate the benefits of moderate sun exposure.

This more balanced view is based on our growing understanding of the benefits of sun-stimulated vitamin D on health. Some major scientific breakthroughs have contributed to this knowledge, and I am proud to have played a part in the discov-

Benefits of Sunlight

- Bone health: Prevents osteoporosis, osteomalacia, and rickets.
- Cellular health: Prevents certain cancers.
- Organ health: Prevents heart disease and stroke.
- Autoimmune health: Prevents multiple sclerosis, Type 1 diabetes mellitus, and rheumatoid arthritis.
- Mood-related health: Prevents seasonal affective disorder, premenstrual tension, and sleeping disorders. It also elevates your sense of well-being (see chapter 5).

ery of some of these advances. Though no media fanfare accompanied publication of the results of the beneficial relationship between sunlight and vitamin D on human health, the news is gradually getting out. The public is finally learning that sunlight and the vitamin D we get from sun exposure is critically important to our health.

The benefits of sunlight on our physical health can be divided into four main areas—bone health, cellular health, organ health, and autoimmune health. There is also the benefit of sunlight on mood-related health (see chapter 5).

Who's at Risk?

People who don't get enough sun exposure are at the greatest risk of being deficient in vitamin D. Older individuals are especially vulnerable. The older you are, the less efficient you

Risk Factors for Vitamin D Deficiency

- **Age.** The older you are, the harder it is for your body to make vitamin D from sunlight.
- **Lifestyle.** The more time you spend indoors during daylight hours, the less opportunity you have to make vitamin D.
- **Geographical location.** If you live in a place with relatively long winters, you get less sun over the course of the year because the sunlight isn't strong enough to make vitamin D in the winter.
- **Race.** People with very dark skin, especially those of African descent, find it difficult to make vitamin D from limited sunlight (their ancestors evolved in a part of the world where sunshine was available year round).
- **Culture.** Certain cultures require that their women cover themselves entirely in heavy clothing that blocks out the sun.

become at making vitamin D from the sun. In fact, your ability to manufacture vitamin D diminishes fourfold from age twenty to age seventy. Senior citizens are especially susceptible to misguided medical advice dispensed through the media. So not only are seniors less efficient at making vitamin D from sunlight, which increases their risk of vitamin D deficiency–related conditions, but they also often exacerbate their situation by going out of their way to avoid sunshine or covering up completely when outdoors in the daytime. The regrettably large number of older Americans who are "shut-ins" are also predisposed to vitamin D deficiency because they receive so little sun exposure.

If you live in a northern climate, you are more likely to be vitamin D deficient because of the relative lack of sunlight available to make vitamin D. A study my colleagues and I recently published showed that 36 percent of healthy white men and women in Boston (medical students and doctors) ages eighteen to twenty-nine were vitamin D deficient at the end of winter. The problem is worse the older you get—42 percent of otherwise healthy Boston-area adults over the age of fifty who participated in the study were found to be vitamin D deficient.

Because melanin is a natural sunscreen, people with darker skin, such as those of African or subcontinental Indian descent, are often vitamin D deficient—especially if they live in northern latitudes or work inside during daylight hours. It takes dark-skinned people significantly longer to make enough vitamin D from sunlight. A dark-skinned person with African lineage may need to spend as much as fifty times longer in the sun to make the same amount of vitamin D as a person of Irish or Scandinavian descent. The U.S. Centers for Disease Control recently reported that throughout the United States, 42 percent of African American women ages fifteen to forty-nine were vitamin D deficient by the end of winter. The situation is worse among elderly people of color. A recent study showed that among the elderly living in the Boston area, 84 percent of African Americans and 42 percent of Hispanics were vitamin D deficient *at the end of summer,* when one would expect vitamin D levels to be at their highest (the figure for elderly Caucasians was a lower but nevertheless alarming 30 percent).

Vitamin D deficiency is seen in other populations as well: young professionals who work indoors; people whose culture

Other Causes of Vitamin D Deficiency

Some people have genetic problems or malfunctions in their kidneys and liver that prevent their bodies from making the active form of vitamin D that benefits health. Here are some of the reasons people may have a vitamin D deficiency even when they get enough sunlight and eat a diet with enough vitamin D in it:

- **Fat malabsorption syndromes.** People whose ability to absorb dietary fat is compromised (fat malabsorption) may need extra vitamin D from sun or tanning bed exposure. Some causes of fat malabsorption are pancreatic enzyme deficiency, Crohn's disease, cystic fibrosis, sprue, liver disease, surgical removal of part or all of the stomach, and small bowel disease. Symptoms of fat malabsorption include diarrhea and greasy and smelly stools.
- **Kidney failure.** Severe kidney disease can interfere with the conversion of 25-vitamin D to activated vitamin D.
- **Vitamin D-dependant rickets (types 1 and 2).** Type 1 affects the body's ability to convert 25-vitamin D to its active form, 1,25-vitamin D, and type 2 interferes with the body's ability to recognize 1,25-vitamin D.
- **Seizure disorders (epilepsy).** Long-term treatment with anticonvulsant medications, such as phenytoin and phenobarbital, can decrease the liver's production of 25-vitamin D.
- **Liver failure.** Liver failure decreases production of 25-vitamin D and makes it difficult for the intestines to absorb vitamin D.

requires them to wear clothing over their entire bodies (such as some Muslim women); people with fat malabsorption conditions (see box above); and breast-fed infants (there is little vitamin D in human milk). Obesity may also predispose you to being vitamin D deficient because body fat is highly efficient at removing vitamin D from the blood (see page 18).

Sunlight and Bone Health

Too often people think of the skeleton as dried up bones mustering in an archaeological dig. In fact, your bones are living things made up of substances that are continually breaking down and being rebuilt. This process is known as "remodeling." Every year, 20 to 40 percent of your skeleton is renewed. Children's bodies make new bone faster than they break down existing bone, which causes bone mass to increase. People reach their peak bone mass in their twenties. However, in the late thirties, the body begins to break down more bone than it makes. This decrease is slight; normal bone loss is only about 0.3 to 0.5 percent per year. The result of this slow loss is that the skeleton becomes less dense and more fragile. The process accelerates the older you get. After menopause, women lose bone density at a rate of 2 to 4 percent every year. Men lose 1 to 2 percent after the age of 60.

If you are trying to ensure the health of your bones, the goal should be to build bone mass when you are young and to maintain it when you get past the age when bone remodeling is at its peak. If you do this, chances are you won't have problems with your bones later in life. But if you don't build bone mass when you are young, and if you lose bone mass at an excessive rate beyond the peak bone building age, your bones can get more porous and brittle, which means they can break more easily (osteoporosis).

If the bone rebuilding process itself is compromised, you may have symptoms such as persistent pain and bone deformity (osteomalacia and rickets).

How can you build bone mass when you are young and maintain it when you are older? The answer to both questions is the same: Be active and get enough calcium in your diet.

When we emphasize calcium intake for bone health, the importance of vitamin D is often ignored. Vitamin D, which you get mostly from the sun, is essential to the process by which you absorb calcium from food and deposit it in your bones. In other words, you can eat as much calcium-rich food as you want to, but if you don't have enough vitamin D in your body, you won't be able to absorb that calcium into your bones. It is estimated that a person who is vitamin D deficient will absorb only about one-third to one-half as much calcium (10 to 15 percent) as he or she would with a healthy vitamin D status (30 percent).

Without enough vitamin D to help your bones absorb calcium—or without enough calcium itself—your bones don't remodel properly. This can happen at any age. Three main bone-related conditions are associated with vitamin D deficiency: osteoporosis, osteomalacia, and, in children, rickets.

Osteoporosis

Bone building depends on a complex series of processes. Crucial among these is the efficient absorption of calcium from the diet. Calcium enters the bloodstream and is deposited in the bones rather like a "cement" to give them their strength. If you are vitamin D deficient, your bones can't get enough calcium, which compromises the bone remodeling process—not enough

What Is Bone Densitometry?

Bone densitometry is a specialized kind of X ray. Bone densitometry calculates how much the X-ray beams are absorbed when passing through bones. The amount of X-ray beams absorbed reveals to doctors the density of the bones being studied. (*Density* refers to the amount of calcium in the bones.) Bone densitometry may be done on the bones of the spine, hip, or wrist. All areas provide similar information because the bone throughout the human body tends to have similar density and usually loses density at the same rate. The result of a densitometry test is known as a "t-score" and is calculated based on how different your bones are from the bone density of a normal young person of your race and gender. A score greater than –2.5 puts you in the category of having osteoporosis.

bone is made to replace the bone that is broken down by parathyroid hormone. This causes bones to become riddled with holes and to become porous, brittle, and weak—a condition known as *osteoporosis*. Vitamin D deficiency can cause osteoporosis, and it can make it worse.

Even when people are consuming enough calcium, numerous studies have shown that they still will not build and maintain bone mass if they are deficient in vitamin D.

Not getting enough vitamin D doesn't just affect your bones in old age. If you don't get enough vitamin D during those early years when it's crucial to build bone mass—up until your thirties—you won't establish the bone mass you need to keep your bones strong when you naturally break down more of the bone structure than you can make.

Men do get osteoporosis, but women are at much greater risk. Women start out with lower bone mass and tend to live longer; they also experience a sudden drop in estrogen at menopause that accelerates bone loss. At the beginning of menopause, women can lose as much as 3 to 4 percent of bone mass every year. Slender, small-framed women are particularly at risk. Men who have low levels of the male hormone testosterone are also at increased risk. Doctors can detect early signs of osteoporosis with a simple, painless bone density test (densitometry).

Not surprisingly, you are at especially high risk of vitamin D deficiency–related osteoporosis if you are predisposed to vitamin D deficiency. Refer to page 78 for information on who's at highest risk for a deficiency in this important vitamin. There is one exception when comparing the risk of vitamin D deficiency and osteoporosis. Although people of African descent living in higher latitudes are at higher risk of vitamin D deficiency because their bodies don't convert sunlight into vitamin D as easily as races with fairer skin, they do *not* appear to be at a higher risk of osteoporosis than those with fairer skin. The reason for this is that people of African genetic lineage tend to start with 7 to 9 percent denser bones than Caucasian people. However, chronic vitamin D deficiency will overcome this natural protection and cause African Americans to suffer increased loss of bone density.

An indication of the importance of vitamin D on the bone density of seniors was found in a study my colleagues and I did of senior citizens living in Maine, which showed that they lose 3 to 4 percent of their bone mass in the fall and winter and regained it in the spring and summer months.

The most serious problem associated with osteoporosis is fractures. Osteoporosis is responsible for 1.5 million fractures

---

Want More Information?

All the studies cited in this book were reviewed by a team of top doctors and published in highly regarded medical journals. References are included at the end of the book. If you want more detailed information on the relationship among sunlight, vitamin D, and health, go to the National Library of Medicine's MEDLINE Web site at www.ncbi.nlm.nih.gov /entrez/query.fcgi and read these studies, and others, for yourself.

---

each year, most notably fractures of the vertebrae (these cause the hunched appearance often seen in elderly women), forearms, wrists, and hips (these are often crippling and sometimes fatal). Osteoporosis-related fractures are more common during the winter months, when bones are less dense due to vitamin D deficiency.

Osteoporosis is known as "the silent threat" because there are no symptoms of pain until a fracture occurs. Numerous studies have shown that vitamin D—usually in conjunction with calcium—is an effective treatment for increasing bone density and preventing fractures associated with osteoporosis. Finnish researchers found that 341 elderly people (mostly women ages seventy-five and older) who were given vitamin D injections experienced fewer fractures than 458 people who did not receive the supplements. A French study of 3,270 elderly women succeeded in reducing hip fractures by 43 percent in participants who were given an 800 IU vitamin D supplement every day compared with those participants who were given a placebo. A study of a less high-risk group was done in the Boston area when

391 men and women ages sixty-five and older were given either a 700 IU vitamin D supplement or a placebo. The results showed that the participants who were given the supplement sustained half as many fractures as the placebo group and experienced significant bone density increases.

Osteomalacia

If you have bone pain and your muscles ache and feel weak, you may have a vitamin D deficiency–related condition called *osteomalacia*. Osteomalacia is frequently described as "softening of the bones." This is slightly misleading. Earlier we described how bones are constantly remodeling—breaking down the old collagen "scaffolding" and building with new material. Osteomalacia is a condition in which the bones don't harden properly during the building phase. A lack of vitamin D is the most common cause of osteomalacia.

Unlike osteoporosis, which is often referred to as a "silent" disease because there are no symptoms until a fracture occurs, the chief characteristic of osteomalacia is severe, unrelenting, deep bone pain. This pain is felt in the bones of the arms, legs, chest, spine, and/or pelvis. Usually there is tenderness of the bones when the doctor pushes down even lightly on the area. The pain from osteomalacia is a result of the unhardened bone matter pressing against the periosteum, which is the nerve-filled fibrous sheath that covers the bones. People with osteomalacia often complain of muscle achiness and weakness.

Osteomalacia is a condition that most severely affects sufferers during the winter months, when lack of vitamin D production is most pronounced.

Is Your "Fibromyalgia" Really Osteomalacia?

Muscle aches, feelings of weakness, and fatigue that just won't quit. Sound familiar? There has been a dramatic increase in various conditions with vague symptoms and no proven way to diagnose them. Among these conditions is fibromyalgia (sometimes known by the names fibrositis, chronic muscle pain syndrome, psychogenic rheumatism, or tension myalgias). Fibromyalgia was unknown until twenty years ago.

The symptoms of fibromyalgia are muscle pain and weakness, though this condition is usually diagnosed when the doctor can't find anything else to explain the vague symptoms of muscle and bone aches. There is no specific test to confirm that a person has fibromyalgia. It is a diagnosis of exclusion. That is, when everything else has been eliminated, this must be what's wrong.

In fact, many people who are told they have fibromyalgia actually have osteomalacia. When someone shows up at a doctor's office with vague symptoms of aching bone pain and muscle weakness, the physician is usually not aware that these are symptoms of vitamin D deficiency. Thus, the patient's vitamin D status is not tested. If it were, doctors would discover that many of the people with these symptoms are vitamin D deficient and they would run specific tests for vitamin D deficiency–related osteomalacia. Between 40 and 60 percent of the people who come to my clinic having been diagnosed with fibromyalgia actually have vitamin D deficiency–related osteomalacia. These patients can be successfully treated with vitamin D supplementation, sunlight, or indoor tanning sessions.

A study of Muslim women living in Denmark who had muscle pain and symptoms consistent with the symptoms of fibromyalgia revealed that 88 percent of them were vitamin D deficient (women in this culture tend to get little sunlight because they spend a lot of time at home and when they go out are obliged to cover themselves entirely).

Often the aching pain associated with osteomalacia is constant and severe. As a result, it can interfere with daily activities and sleep. Muscle weakness is also common and comes and goes unexpectedly. This pain can increase the risk of injuries from falling. If you have osteomalacia that continues unabated, it will weaken your bones and predispose you to fractures, especially of the lower spine, hip, and wrist.

How do we test for osteomalacia? X-rays and bone density tests aren't effective diagnostic tools because they cannot distinguish between osteomalacia and osteoporosis. If my patient complains of the characteristic symptoms of this condition and a physical examination reveals bone pain when I press down lightly on the breastbone (sternum), the outside of the shin of the lower leg, and the forearms, then I will diagnose that person with vitamin D deficiency–related osteomalacia and initiate intensive oral vitamin D therapy (an eight-week course of 50,000 IU doses of vitamin D once a week), including moderate sun exposure in spring, summer, and fall. To confirm the diagnosis, I will order a blood test to measure the serum level of 25-vitamin D, which is an accurate gauge of a person's vitamin D status. After two months, I will test the patient's blood again to make sure the vitamin D deficiency has been corrected. Usually the therapy I prescribe resolves the condition. If not, I prescribe another eight-week course of oral vitamin D once a week. It can take months or years to develop osteomalacia, and it may take just as long to overcome this condition.

Rickets (Pediatric Osteomalacia)

In fully grown adults, no matter how bad the pain, there are no visible symptoms of osteomalacia. In children whose bones are still growing, however, bones that don't harden properly may bend under the weight of the child's body—a condition known as "rickets" or pediatric osteomalacia. Typical signs of rickets include legs that bend inward or outward or a sunken chest with rivetlike bone protrusions up and down both sides of the breast. The ends of the bones of the arms and legs may be wider than normal. In addition to these visible deformities, children with rickets experience bone pain and muscle weakness.

Rickets was first identified in Europe in the mid-1600s, and it became a major problem during the Industrial Revolution. Doctors of the era were dismayed to find widespread bone deformation in urban youngsters that was unknown in European farm kids or even the poorest children of Asia and Africa. Dr. Jedrzej Sniadecki of Poland determined that rickets was caused by lack of sunlight. European cities were a maze of dark alleyways where the sun did not penetrate, and overhead the skies were clouded with heavy pollution. Furthermore, many children of this period were forced to work all day in factories.

It wasn't until the 1920s that Doctors Alfred Hess and Lester Unger—based on Dr. Sniadecki's research—demonstrated that sunlight could be used to cure rickets. As a result, countless numbers of children were cured of rickets simply by exposing them to the sunshine. Boston's famed Floating Hospital was originally a large boat that took city children with vitamin D deficiency into Boston Harbor, where they could sit above decks to be exposed to the sun.

Until the 1930s, sunlight was the treatment for rickets (artificial sunlight from mercury arc lamps was also used). When scientists discovered it was possible to fortify milk with vitamin D and governments in Europe and North America sanctioned

What My Family's Pet Iguana Taught Me

The Holick family iguana is called Raptor, and he and other reptiles provide dramatic insight into the importance of UVB radiation on bone health. In nature, reptiles continually bathe in the sun to warm their cold-blooded bodies as well as to make vitamin D to strengthen their bones. When in captivity, reptiles have difficulty getting any sun to ensure their bone health because they live in an enclosed environment. Young pet reptiles often have rickets, and older ones have osteoporosis. As a result, even the most benign of accidents—such as falling off a perch—can lead to bone fractures. When X-rayed, many captive reptiles are found to have multiple fractures, which often lead to their death.

Responsible and educated reptile owners now understand it is essential to install UVB lamps in their pets' enclosures. Doing this effectively prevents the kinds of fractures previously seen in captive reptiles because it results in much stronger, denser bones.

This phenomenon is identical to what human bodies experience when they do not get enough UVB exposure—a weakening of the bones that results in unnecessary fractures.

In addition to my work in the field of how sunshine affects human health, I enjoy a degree of renown for improving the health of four-legged residents of planet earth. I am helping develop lighting for reptile enclosures that replicates natural sunshine, and I advise the staffs of the National Zoo, the San Diego Zoo, and the Cleveland Zoo on how to keep their indoor reptiles healthy.

the fortification of milk and other foods with vitamin D, rickets was effectively eradicated. However, in the 1950s, unregulated vitamin D fortification in the United Kingdom resulted in a slew of cases of vitamin D intoxication in infants. Therefore,

European governments passed laws prohibiting the fortification of milk with this vitamin. As a result, rickets has again become a significant health problem in children living in cramped European urban communities such as London, Glasgow, and Paris.

The United States may be poised for a resurgence of rickets. Already sporadic cases are appearing. Because the disease has become so rare and doctors are not required by law to report it, however, no national statistics are available. The main reasons for the reemergence of this condition are the increase in breast-feeding infants (human milk contains almost no vitamin D) and the decline in young children's exposure to natural sunlight. Breast-feeding is important for a child's health, but it is important that both infant and mother take a vitamin D supplement.

Although the incidence of rickets among American children is still extremely low, it is a growing problem. Parents need to be vigilant about their children's diet and lifestyle.

The foundation of treatment for rickets is restoring the child's vitamin D status. Bracing, and sometimes surgery, may be necessary to correct skeletal deformities that have occurred.

Preventing Bone Conditions Related to Vitamin D Deficiency

Preventing bone disorders caused by a deficiency in vitamin D is quite straightforward. To keep them from getting rickets, make sure that your children get plenty of calcium and vitamin D in their diets and that they spend some time outdoors without sun protection. Playing outdoors for a short time does not require the use of sunscreens, but anytime there is the risk of a burn, you should make sure your child wears a high-SPF broad-spectrum sunscreen. Exercise in childhood is also important, as it increases the bone density that is essential in later life.

As adults, you also need to eat a diet rich in calcium and vitamin D, and you need to exercise. Strength training with weights can be especially effective at building strong bones. And yes, it's important that you make use of that fantastic all-natural source of vitamin D—the sun. Just a few minutes of unprotected sun exposure on your face, hands, and arms (or arms and legs) on sunny days is enough for most people. Exactly how much sun exposure you need depends on a variety of factors, including your skin type, where you live, and how often you can get out in the sun. Chapter 7 provides specific information on how to measure the sun exposure you need.

Treating Vitamin D Related Bone Conditions

If you have a bone condition caused by vitamin D deficiency, then your vitamin D "tank" is empty and needs to be filled as quickly as possible. Sun exposure for only a few days and over-the-counter supplements in pill form usually aren't effective enough.

If I diagnose someone with a bone condition whose blood test reveals she is vitamin D deficient (the 25-vitamin D in her blood is less than 20 ng/ml; 1/50,000 of a gram in 1 gram of blood—see figure 4.1), then I will prescribe an intensive program to restore her vitamin D level, generally consisting of 50,000 IU of vitamin D weekly for eight weeks. This can only be prescribed by a doctor. Although the patient's 25-vitamin D level will go up quickly, the symptoms related to vitamin D de-

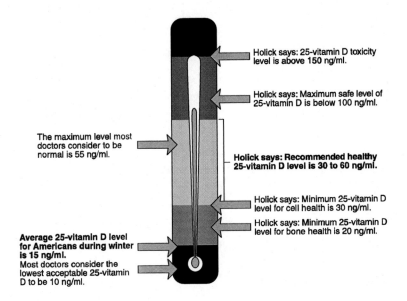

The maximum level most doctors consider to be normal is 55 ng/ml.

Average 25-vitamin D level for Americans during winter is 15 ng/ml.
Most doctors consider the lowest acceptable 25-vitamin D to be 10 ng/ml.

Holick says: 25-vitamin D toxicity level is above 150 ng/ml.

Holick says: Maximum safe level of 25-vitamin D is below 100 ng/ml.

Holick says: Recommended healthy 25-vitamin D level is 30 to 60 ng/ml.

Holick says: Minimum 25-vitamin D level for cell health is 30 ng/ml.

Holick says: Minimum 25-vitamin D level for bone health is 20 ng/ml.

Figure 4.1 Holick barometer of vitamin D status

ficiency may take several weeks or months to lessen, and many months to resolve completely.

Sun exposure is just as effective a way to build a person's vitamin D level. If you sunbathe in a bathing suit on the beach or in your backyard, you will have received a dose of between 10,000 and 25,000 IU of vitamin D when you are slightly pink (1MED). This slight pinkness is a sign of a mild burn, and I always discourage anyone from getting a burn. Instead, spending *one-quarter* of the amount of time in the sun that it takes you to get pink is the safest way to build your vitamin D levels, and doing this three times a week will provide you with weekly dosage of vitamin D equivalent to 15,000 IU. This amount of sun exposure is usually enough to correct a vitamin D deficiency. If

A Quick Look at the Holick Formula for Safe Sun

The Holick Formula for Safe Sun is a guide to how much sun exposure you need to maintain appropriate vitamin D levels. Here's how it works.

Estimate how long it will take for you to get a mild sunburn (when your skin gets pink—known as 1MED), then two to three times a week, expose your face, hands, and arms (or arms and legs) for 20 to 25 percent of that time. In other words, if it would take thirty minutes for your skin to get pink in the sunshine (as it would for me at noon on a Cape Cod beach in the summertime), then two to three times a week spend six to eight minutes in the sun before putting on SPF15 sunscreen. Always adjust your calculations depending on the situation. For example, if you are at the beach at ten in the morning or four in the afternoon, the sun is less strong, so you can spend longer in the sun without protection (if you estimate that at that time, based on your experience, it would take an hour for you to get a 1MED, then you can spend about fifteen minutes in the sun without any sunscreen on). Remember, I do not advocate that you ever get a mild sunburn, but simply that you estimate how long it would take you to get a 1MED and make your calculations of safe sun time accordingly.

you work during the day, an indoor tanning facility can provide the same benefits.

Sunlight and Cellular Health

Doctors have long understood that sun deprivation causes bone problems, but only relatively recently has the connection been made between sunshine and the decreased risk of a variety of cellular health conditions, such as internal cancers, especially

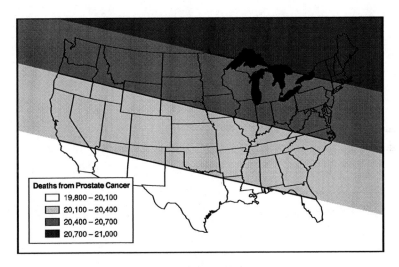

Figure 4.2 *Cancer rates and UVB availability.* This map shows the rates of prostate cancer in different regions of the United States. According to Hanchette and Schwartz (1992), the sunnier the region, the fewer prostate deaths there are. The same trend has been identified in analyses of breast and colon cancer rates. (Source: National Cancer Institute)

those that affect the breast, colon, and prostate. Increasingly, epidemiologists (doctors who study the cause and transmission of diseases within populations) are discovering that people who live in sunnier climates have a lower incidence of these killer diseases than people who live in climates where there are limited amounts of sunlight.

One of the first doctors to identify the connection between how much sun people get throughout the year and their risk of disease was Dr. Frank Apperly. In the early 1940s, he observed that people who live in sunny climates have a lower risk of cancer than people who lived in climates with less sunlight (see figure 4.2). Apperly analyzed cancer statistics throughout North America and Canada. Compared with cities at a latitude of between 10 and 30 degrees, cities between 30 and 40 degrees latitude averaged 85 percent higher overall cancer death rates, cities between 40 and 50 degrees latitude averaged 118 percent higher cancer death rates, and cities between 50 and 60 degrees latitude averaged 150 percent higher cancer death rates.

Numerous studies have since confirmed Apperly's findings. A 1990 study published in *Preventive Medicine* showed that women living in the sunnier southwest of the United States were only about half as likely to die from breast cancer as were women in the least sunny northeast region of the country. A 1992 article in *Preventive Medicine* analyzing fifty years of epidemiological cancer data suggested that increasing sun exposure would reduce the number of breast and colon cancer deaths by 30,000, or one-third. In 2001, *Lancet* published an article that directly linked sun exposure to decreased prostate cancer rates. This study showed that British people who got sunburned as children, who vacationed in sunny countries, and who made a habit of sunbathing were much less likely to develop prostate cancer. They also found that people who spent lots of time in the sun tended to develop prostate cancer later than those who spent little time in the sun (at an average of 67.7 years old as compared to 72.1 years). Because prostate cancer grows very slowly, this five-year delay in the age of diagnosis is highly significant.

Two major studies published in 2002 reinforced the link between sunlight and cancer prevention. Doctors from the National Cancer Institute reported that people who either worked outdoors or who lived in sunny climates were less likely to die from breast or colon cancer. They also found that the risk of dying from cancers of the ovaries and prostate were lower among people living nearer the equator. In the journal *Cancer* a month earlier, a researcher described how sunlight was responsible for preventing a range of cancers of the reproductive and digestive system. The study's author, Dr. William Grant, revealed how, compared with residents of the Southwest, people in New England were twice as likely to develop cancers of the breast, ovaries, colon, prostate, bladder, uterus, esophagus, rectum, and stomach. Based on the statistics available, Grant calculates that in 2002 alone insufficient sun exposure among Americans caused 85,000 more cases of cancer and 30,000 more deaths than if everyone in the United States got as much sun as people living in the Southwest. Similar observations have been made in Europe.

You may ask, What about the increased rates of melanoma and non-melanoma skin cancer that would hypothetically result from this additional sun exposure? Grant calculates the additional number of deaths from skin cancer would be 3,000—a tragically high number, but one far smaller than the number of deaths caused by *underexposure* to sunlight.

Certain types of cancer have strong gender associations. Breast cancer affects mostly women, and only men get prostate cancer. Both breast and prostate cancer are strongly influenced by sun exposure.

Breast Cancer

In the United States, about 50,000 women die from breast cancer every year—making it the deadliest killer of women after heart disease. To the more than 180,000 women who are diagnosed with this disease, there are not only physical consequences but emotional ones too. Self-esteem issues associated with breast cancer can be profound.

In May 1999, a landmark study led by Dr. Ester John, based on the meticulous analysis of breast cancer statistics from the National Health and Nutrition Examination Survey, was published. The results provide extraordinary insight into the relationship between sun exposure and breast cancer. The authors conclude definitively that sun exposure and a vitamin D-rich diet significantly lower the risk of breast cancer.

The John study demonstrates that increased sun exposure alone could potentially reduce the incidence and death rate of breast cancer in the United States by 35 to 75 percent. This would mean that the incidence of new cases might be reduced by 70,000 to 150,000 each year and that 17,500 to 37,500 deaths could be prevented. A conservative estimate is that increased sun exposure could prevent 100,000 new cases of breast cancer and 27,500 deaths from this disease. Combining increased sun exposure with a vitamin D-rich diet or supplements could make the disease prevention and death rate figures 150,000 and 37,500, respectively. Based on his studies, Dr. Grant estimates that lack of sun exposure is responsible for approximately 25 percent of the deaths from breast cancer in Europe.

It is difficult to imagine the excitement that would result if a drug were invented that yielded such results!

What about skin cancer rates? Wouldn't they rise in response to increased sun exposure? Approximately 500 women a year die from non-melanoma skin cancer. Given that the above statistics show that 27,500 women die prematurely because of *underexposure* to sunlight, it becomes evident that 55 women die prematurely because of *underexposure* to sunlight for every 1 who dies prematurely from *overexposure* to sunlight.

Prostate Cancer

Only heart attacks and lung cancer kill more men than cancer of the prostate, which every year claims more than 50,000 lives in the United States alone.

Prostate cancer kills 1 in 4 men who get this disease, making it one of the most deadly forms of cancer. By comparison, you have a 1 in 7 chance of dying from melanoma, a 1 in 800 chance of dying from non-melanoma skin cancer, and a 1 in 2,600 chance of dying from basal cell carcinoma, which makes up 80 percent of all non-melanoma skin cancers. About 40,000 American men die every year from prostate cancer—more than ten times as many as are killed by melanomas.

Cancer of the prostate is especially feared by men because surgical treatment for this form of cancer frequently results in impotence. A study in the August 2001 issue of *Lancet* proves that the risk of developing prostate cancer is directly related to sunlight exposure. The study divided people into four groups according to how much sunlight they had been exposed to. The lowest quarter of the study participants, or quartile, were three times more likely to develop prostate cancer than those in the highest quartile of sun exposure. The results show that those in the highest quartile reduced their risk of developing prostate cancer by 66 percent. Those in the second and third quartiles also had a significantly lower chance of getting prostate cancer compared with those in the lowest quartile, who received the least amount of sun exposure.

Only about 600 men die prematurely each year from non-melanoma skin cancer, but 37,000 men die prematurely each

---

Hypertension: The Silent Killer

One in four adult Americans—50 million in all—suffers from hypertension, the main sign of which is high blood pressure. More than half of Americans more than sixty years old have hypertension. Despite its prevalence, high blood pressure is often ignored or undiagnosed because it has no symptoms. However, hypertension is a prime risk factor for heart disease and stroke, the first and third leading causes of death in this country. Because it is an insidious and deadly disease, hypertension is sometimes called "the silent killer."

---

year from prostate cancer. It's possible to conclude that 55 to 60 men die prematurely from *underexposure* to sunlight for every 1 that dies prematurely due to *overexposure*. Even when you include melanoma—for which sunshine is only one of several risk factors—the numbers are still lopsided: about 10 to 1.

Colon Cancer

Cancer of the colon and its neighboring area, known sometimes as colorectal cancer, affects both men and women. Like breast cancer and prostate cancer, colorectal cancer is seen much more frequently than skin cancers and is much more deadly. According to the Garland studies, you are three times less likely to die from colon cancer if you have healthy levels of 25-vitamin D in your blood stream (20 ng/ml or more).

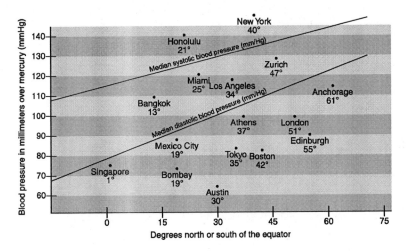

Figure 4.3 The farther you live from the equator (and therefore the less available sun there is to make vitamin D), the higher your blood pressure is likely to be. (Source: Rostand)

Sunlight and Organ Health

Sun exposure has an equally dramatic effect on heart and circulatory disease. High blood pressure, also known as hypertension, is a very serious condition that is the main cause of stroke and heart attack. If you live in a sunny climate, you are less likely to have high blood pressure than if you live somewhere with less sunlight at certain times of the year. In fact, the farther away from the equator you live, the higher your blood pressure gets (see figure 4.3). People tend to have healthier blood pressure during the summer than winter because there's more sunlight available. When exposed to the same amount of sunlight, people with fairer skin have healthier blood pressure than those with dark skin (the darker your skin, the more melanin there is in it, and consequently the more difficult it is for you to produce vitamin D from the sun). There's now specific evidence that people who live in sunnier climates have fewer heart attacks. Heart failure is also associated with vitamin D deficiency.

How Science Proved Vitamin D Is Good for Cellular and Organ Health

When epidemiologists ruled out other factors that might explain the better cellular and organ health of people who live in sunnier climates—such as diet, exercise, and alcohol and tobacco use—the search was on to discover the connection between sunshine and decreased risk of certain common diseases. Those of us in the vitamin D field felt sure there was a connection between this important vitamin and good health. As it turned out, we were right!

Vitamin D and Cellular Health

Toward the end of the 1980s, I was part of a small but growing movement of medical scientists who believed that the active form of vitamin D that I had discovered a decade earlier had benefits well beyond bone health. We theorized that people who lived in sunnier climates had lower rates of cancer and heart disease because the vitamin D produced by their exposure to the sun was somehow benefiting cells throughout the body. A few studies backed this up, but what exactly was happening to cause this?

There was profound disagreement on the subject, and I respectfully declined to have my name appear on published articles, even when my laboratory did the vitamin D analysis for the study. My fellow researchers had successfully proved the relationship between sunlight and cellular health, but I believed their conclusion as to *why* sunlight and increased vitamin D production benefited cellular health was incorrect. They thought that vitamin D benefited cells throughout the body in the same way we understood it benefited bone health. That is, the more sunshine you get, the more 25-vitamin D there is circulating in your bloodstream that can be converted by the kidneys into activated vitamin D. According to this theory, this activated vitamin D would then be sent by the kidneys to different parts of the body where it would benefit different cell groups (refer to figure 1.2). This theory assumes that the more vitamin D you get from the sun and diet, the more activated vitamin D your kidneys will make.

I believed something quite different. My theory was considered heretical (and would still be thought of this way if my colleagues and I hadn't proved it). We understood that activated vitamin D is one of the most potent inhibitors of abnormal cell growth, but we knew that no matter how much you increased the supply of 25-vitamin D in a person's body through sunlight and diet, you couldn't get the kidneys to make any more activated vitamin D from it. I didn't think the very limited amount of activated vitamin D the kidneys are able to produce could be responsible for all the cellular benefits that had been identified. *There had to be another source of activated vitamin D*, or so I believed.

What my colleagues and I proposed was that cells throughout the body don't have to rely on the meager supply of activated vitamin D from the kidneys because they each have their own enzymatic machinery to convert 25-vitamin D into activated vitamin D (refer to figure 1.3).

We proved this theory in a study published in 1998. Our findings completely changed the way medical science perceives the relationship between vitamin D and cellular and organ health. What we did in this study was expose prostate cancer cells to 25-vitamin D to see what would happen. In cancerous fashion, these cells were reproducing out of control. When we exposed these prostate cancer cells to 25-vitamin D, they converted that substance into activated vitamin D and the cells stopped their chaotic reproduction. What we had actually *proven* was that, just like the kidney, prostate cancer cells could make activated vitamin D. But unlike the activated vitamin D made by the kidneys, which regulates calcium metabolism and promotes bone health, the activated vitamin D created within the prostate has the specific job of ensuring healthy cell growth. Not only was this confirmed in subsequent studies, but also similar studies by my research group and other researchers found that the same enzymatic machinery to activate vitamin D also exists in the cells of the colon and breast.

The consequences of this discovery are mind-boggling. We had discovered the likely reason why sun exposure has such a profound effect on cancer rates. When you are exposed to more sunlight and make more vitamin D, it can be converted by the liver into 25-vitamin D, which can be activated by the prostate, colon, ovaries, breast, and probably most other tissues to prevent unhealthy cell growth. The more you make, the healthier these disease-prone tissues will be.

Because we don't have to rely on a supply of activated vitamin D from our kidneys, there is an enormous capacity to treat cancer with powerful new synthetic forms of activated vitamin D. Studies are now under way in humans (we proved it works in mice), and the potential is enormous.

Vitamin D and Organ Health

What about cardiovascular health? Scientists now believe that the work we did on activated vitamin D also has a bearing on those cells important to heart and circulatory health, especially the blood vessels. Blood vessels are the tubular channels—the arteries and veins—through which blood circulates throughout your body. High blood pressure can occur if the blood vessels get stiff and narrow, which increases the pressure inside them. The work showing that there are vitamin D receptors in various cells throughout the body and that these cells activate vitamin D led me and other scientists to conclude that there are also vitamin D receptors in the cells of our blood vessels. The effect of vitamin D on the blood vessels is to make them relax and be more flexible. It does this by lessening the effects of the renin-angiotensin system on the blood vessels. The blood flows more smoothly through them, and there is less pressure against the blood pressure walls.

I have participated in several studies to investigate the effects of UVB on heart health. My colleagues and I have found that regularly exposing patients with high blood pressure to UVB in a tanning bed causes their blood pressure to become normal—in other words, they get healthier. The best known of these studies was published in *Lancet*. In this study, we showed that exposing patients to UVB in a tanning bed three times a week for six weeks elevated bloodstream 25-vitamin D by 162 percent and reduced diastolic blood pressure by 6 mmHg and systolic blood pressure by 6 mmHg. (That's about as much as certain blood pressure medications do but without the unpleasant side effects!) How did we know that the UVB was at work rather than the warmth and relaxing environment affecting this change? We provided the same treatments to a separate set of patients using a UVA tanning bed, and this made no difference to vitamin D levels or blood pressure. For the entire nine months we followed them, those patients who continued with the tanning bed treatments maintained a healthier, lower blood pressure. Remember that high blood pressure is one of the leading causes of death in the United States and the rest of the industrialized world because it is a main cause of heart attack and stroke.

My colleagues and I studied areas of heart health other than hypertension. To confirm the pioneering work of Dr. Malte Bühring and Dr. Rolfdeiter Krause, I was part of a team of researchers who exposed a group of heart disease patients to UVB three times a week for a month. Increasing 25-vitamin D levels in the body in this way improved heart health in a variety of ways—heart strength was increased (as measured by blood-pumping ability), and heart strain was decreased (as measured by resting and nonresting heart rate and the accumulation of lactic acid). Our studies and other research teams' efforts show that the benefits of UVB on heart health are similar to those of an exercise program. When *combined* with physical fitness, UVB exposure has been shown to have extremely beneficial results.

The results of the studies to treat heart and circulatory health with UVB radiation demonstrate why people who spend time in the sun tend to have healthier blood pressure levels and better all around heart health.

What can *you* do to prevent cancer and improve your heart and circulatory health? Of course it's important to do all the things you've heard before—don't smoke, eat healthfully, and be physically active. In addition, make sure you spend enough time in the sun to maintain appropriate 25-vitamin D levels.

Sunlight and Autoimmune Diseases

The immune system protects the body by defending it against invading microorganisms, such as viruses and bacteria. It does this by producing antibodies or particular kinds of white blood cells, called *sensitized lymphocytes*, to attack these unwelcome invaders. If your immune system is working as it should, it won't attack fellow cells; it will only respond to threats from trespassers. But if something goes wrong, your immune system may malfunction and signal antibodies and sensitized lymphocytes to attack your own cells. This usually occurs because of an external disturbance to your immune system from a medication, bacteria, or virus combined with a genetic predisposition to autoimmune disease.

Among the most common diseases associated with the autoimmune system are multiple sclerosis, Type 1 diabetes, rheumatoid arthritis, and psoriasis (although there is some controversy as to whether psoriasis is actually an autoimmune disease—I don't believe it is).

For some time, epidemiologists have known that autoimmune diseases are less common in regions close to the equator, where there is more sunshine throughout the year. As was recently discovered, one of the main reasons for this may be that because immune cells have vitamin D receptors (VDRs), they may benefit from the vitamin D the body generates from sun exposure. As stated earlier in this chapter, vitamin D also promotes other areas of cellular health, which makes it less likely that an undesirable autoimmune response will occur. Thus, sun exposure is an effective preventive measure against autoimmune diseases. Therefore, activated vitamin D and artificial forms of this substance (known as activated vitamin D analogs) are increasingly being tested as a therapy for diseases that have an autoimmune component.

Multiple Sclerosis

Multiple sclerosis (MS) is a chronic, debilitating disease that affects the brain and spinal cord, which together make up the central nervous system. In MS, your body sends immune cells to the brain and spinal cord that result in nerve damage to these structures. Eventually, multiple areas of scarring (sclerosis) develop, causing slowed or blocked muscle coordination and weakness, double vision, and eventually loss of sight and other nerve signals. Most people develop MS between the ages of twenty and forty. An estimated 330,000 Americans have MS, and there are thought to be 2.5 million sufferers worldwide. The disease is twice as common in women as in men.

There is a well-established genetic component in MS—if someone in your family had the disease, you are much more likely to get it. About 20 percent of people with MS have at least one affected relative. If you're a first-degree relative of someone with MS, such as a child or a sibling, your chance of eventually developing MS is twenty to forty times greater than if you aren't.

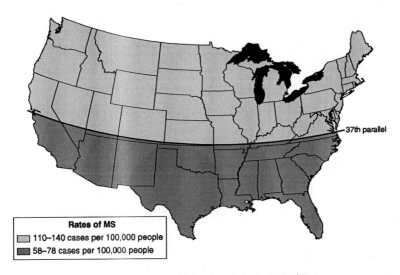

Figure 4.4 Rates of multiple sclerosis in the United States
are higher above the 37th parallel.

There is also an undisputed connection between sun exposure and MS. The disease is about five times more likely to affect
you if you live in North America or Europe compared with the
tropics. In the United States, MS is far more prevalent in states
above the 37th parallel than in states below it (see figure 4.4).
From east to west, the 37th parallel extends from Newport
News, Virginia, to Santa Cruz, California, and runs along the
northern border of North Carolina to the northern border of
Arizona, including most of California. The MS prevalence rate
for the region below the 37th parallel is 57 to 78 cases per
100,000 people. The prevalence rate for those above the 37th
parallel is almost double that: 110 to 140 cases per 100,000
people. Early sun exposure is key—fifteen years old seems to be
the cutoff age at which where you grew up determines the likelihood that you will develop MS. In other words, if you grew up in

the tropics and moved to a country in the northern latitudes after age fifteen, your risk of developing MS stays low, and conversely if you grew up in the northern latitudes and moved to the tropics, you would continue to have a higher risk of developing MS.

Even though their risk of MS goes down if they move to a sunny climate, Scandinavians and Celtic people of northern Europe appear to be predisposed to MS wherever they are. As a result of generations of sun deprivation, these populations may have a higher risk of MS because their immune system has, in certain cases, been genetically altered. Based on epidemiological studies, scientists reason that it probably has something to do with a lack of vitamin D from sunlight that caused the immune system of some people living in these northern latitudes to go awry and attack the nervous system. Confirmation of this theory is found in studies showing that Norwegians who live near the coast and eat a diet high in vitamin D-rich foods have a much lower risk of MS than those who live inland. Because they live in high latitudes, both groups are at risk of not getting enough natural sunlight. On the other hand, there is almost no incidence of MS among Eskimos who live in very high latitudes. This is thought to be because of their traditional vitamin D-rich diet of polar bear liver, whale and seal blubber, and oily fish.

We know that immune cells have vitamin D receptors. When these cells are exposed to appropriate amounts of activated vitamin D, some of which is made by the immune cells themselves, they respond by doing the job they should do and not launching attacks against the body they are supposed to protect. A group led by Dr. Hector DeLuca used lab studies to demonstrate that pretreating mice with activated vitamin D and then trying to trigger the autoimmune response that causes MS (as it is possible to do) resulted in no MS symptoms. This was due to the protective effect of the activated vitamin D.

Unfortunately, despite the tantalizing possibility that vitamin D may be the key to treating MS, so far doctors haven't been able to develop an activated vitamin D therapy that effectively slows or halts the progression of the disease in humans (although vitamin D is successfully used to treat some of the muscle and bone pain caused by vitamin D deficiency in people with MS). Part of the problem is that by the time a person is diagnosed with MS, it's too late to reverse the autoimmune process that causes the nerve damage. Researchers are testing different ways of administering large doses of activated vitamin D to people with MS, but the results have been disappointing. We're still holding out hope that one day we will develop a method of treating MS with activated vitamin D that can help the millions of people worldwide who have this devastating disease.

Until then, it is reasonable to suggest that you can lessen your own and your children's risk of developing MS by getting enough sun exposure to build appropriate levels of vitamin D and, failing that, taking a supplement with enough vitamin D in it to meet all your minimum daily needs (refer to chapter 7 for guidelines). This is especially important if you grew up in the northern latitudes or are of Scandinavian or Celtic heritage.

Type 1 Diabetes (Juvenile Diabetes/ Insulin-Dependant Diabetes Mellitus)

Type 1 diabetes is a chronic disease that occurs when the beta islet cells of the pancreas, which are responsible for making insulin, are attacked and eventually destroyed by the immune system. This condition is different from Type 2, or "adult onset," diabetes, which occurs in adulthood and is not a disease of the immune system. In Type 1 diabetes, the pancreas can't produce enough insulin to regulate blood sugar levels and eventually can't produce any insulin at all because all the beta islet cells have been destroyed. This disease almost always occurs in childhood. Without enough insulin, glucose builds up in the bloodstream instead of entering the cells. The body then can't use the glucose for energy despite high levels in the bloodstream. This causes symptoms such as excessive thirst, frequent need to urinate, and hunger. Five to ten years after the onset of diabetes, the beta islet cells are destroyed and the pancreas is unable to make any insulin at all. Severe diseases, including blindness, kidney failure, hypertension, and heart disease, are among the regrettable complications of end-stage diabetes. Circulation may deteriorate to the extent that ulcers on the legs don't heal, and amputations of the foot or legs may be necessary.

People who live in sunny climates tend to have lower risks of diabetes. This disease is very rare in equatorial regions. Conversely, regions with limited amounts of sunlight have a higher incidence of diabetes. Northern Finns experience only two hours of sunlight on December days, and Finland has the world's highest reported incidence of Type 1 diabetes.

Activated vitamin D may help prevent Type 1 diabetes by making the beta islet cells more resistant to attack from the immune system and by enhancing insulin output by these cells. It can also improve the health of the immune system, making it less likely that it will malfunction and attack the beta islet cells in the first place. Although epidemiological studies have long suggested that vitamin D from sun exposure provides immunity to diabetes, a recent study done in Finland rocked the medical establishment and confirmed what many of us believed about the relationship between vitamin D and this disease. The study followed more than 12,000 babies born in 1966. Those who were given a vitamin D supplement had an 80 percent reduced risk of developing diabetes compared with babies who did not receive a supplement. Recent research shows that UVB radiation may have a role in preventing Type 2, or "adult onset," diabetes, because activated vitamin D can increase insulin production.

What does all this information mean? What should you do to reduce your own and your children's risk of developing Type 1 diabetes? The studies reinforce the need to get appropriate amounts of sun exposure. During the summertime, your kids need to spend time outdoors—not sitting on the couch watching TV or playing video games. Refer to chapter 7 for specific guidelines on how much sun is needed for optimal vitamin D health.

Rheumatoid Arthritis

Rheumatoid arthritis (RA) is a chronic inflammatory disease that primarily affects the joints, but it can also affect other organ systems. Although the disease can strike a person at any age, it usually comes on between the ages of twenty-five and fifty-five. The disease is more common in older people. Women are affected almost three times as often as men. Between 1 and 2 percent of Americans have RA. The rate of advance and severity of the illness varies a great deal from person to person.

Symptoms of Rheumatoid Arthritis

The areas of the body most commonly affected by rheumatoid arthritis are the wrists, knees, elbows, fingers, toes, ankles, and neck. Individuals with RA experience bilateral joint pain, joint stiffness, joint warmth, and joint swelling. Here are some other common symptoms to watch for:

- Fatigue
- Discomfort
- Appetite loss
- Mild fever
- Morning stiffness for more than one hour
- Joint deformities in the hands and feet
- Round, painless nodules under the skin
- Skin redness or inflammation
- Eye irritation and discharge
- Numbness and/or tingling

When a person gets RA, the immune system attacks the lining of the joints, a substance known as *synovium*, which then becomes inflamed. Wrists, fingers, knees, feet, and ankles are the joints most commonly affected. The process is usually "bilateral," which means it effects both knees, both wrists, and so on. Symptoms include pain, swelling, and stiffness of the joints that can lead to joint deformity. These symptoms distinguish rheumatoid arthritis from osteoarthritis, which is a more common and degenerative "wear-and-tear" arthritis.

Complications of RA can be very severe and may include joint destruction, heart failure, lung disease, anemia, low or high platelets, eye disease, cervical (neck) spine instability, neuropathy, and vasculitis.

There are no known ways to prevent RA, although the disease's progression can be slowed with early detection and aggressive treatment. Current treatment focuses on reducing inflammation of the joints with anti-inflammatory or immunosuppressive medications such as prednisone, methotrexate, and Enbrel.

Unfortunately, most of the successful pharmacological treatments have serious side effects, from life-threatening gastrointestinal bleeding to osteoporosis. Infections also may occur due to the suppression of the immune system. Millions upon millions of dollars are being spent to develop effective treatments for RA that do not have serious side effects.

Scientists began testing the effects of vitamin D on rheumatoid arthritis in the 1940s, but initial overdoses caused testing to be suspended until renewed interest began in the 1990s. Why this renewed interest? We now understand much better the role of activated vitamin D on cellular health. In addition, we have much more efficient and safer ways of administering vitamin D treatment. Both developments make it reasonable to revisit the prospect of using vitamin D to treat RA.

Preliminary studies show that vitamin D is indeed an effective treatment for RA. Mice with RA that were given activated vitamin D experienced a diminishment of the cellular activity responsible for this immune disease, giving rise to the expectation that there may come a day when we can successfully treat RA with injections of activated vitamin D or oral activated vitamin D pills.

Psoriasis

Plaque psoriasis is a chronic skin disease that humankind has known about for millennia (the word *psoriasis* is the ancient Greek word for "itch"). Today this disease affects 5.5 million people in the United States and 50 million people worldwide. The condition mostly affects adults, and the symptoms can be extremely distressing, both physically and psychologically.

The characteristic symptoms of psoriasis are raised patches of thick, red skin covered with silvery scales. These unsightly patches, sometimes called "plaques," generally itch and may burn. Psoriasis usually occurs on the elbows, knees, scalp, lower back, face, palms, and soles of the feet, but it can affect skin anywhere on the body. In areas such as the knees and elbows, the skin may crack. The disease sometimes affects the fingernails, the toenails, and the flesh inside the mouth. About 15 percent of people with psoriasis have joint inflammation, which produces a crippling form of arthritis called psoriatic arthritis.

Under normal circumstances, skin cells grow, divide, and replace themselves in an orderly fashion, but with psoriasis, cells start reproducing out of control. Psoriatic skin may "turn over" (be replaced) in as little as four days, compared with normal skin, which turns over in twenty-eight days. This rapid turnover, combined with altered maturation of skin cells, results in the characteristic symptoms of psoriasis.

Long before doctors established that psoriasis would benefit from directed vitamin D therapy, people with psoriasis knew that their condition improved in response to sun exposure. Folk remedies for psoriasis invariably included sun baths.

One of the first modern medical breakthroughs in treating psoriasis with UV radiation was made in the 1920s by the German doctor William Goeckermann. Goeckermann theorized that, because sunlight helped lessen the symptoms of psoriasis, increasing the intensity of the sun's radiation on the skin of a person who had psoriasis could increase the healthy effects of the sun. Goeckermann applied a solution of coal tar to the affected areas of skin and then subjected those areas to the radiation of a sunlamp. The coal tar did indeed intensify the effect of the sun's radiation and reduced the symptoms of psoriasis even more than did UV radiation alone.

Versions of Goeckermann's treatment of psoriasis are still used today by many dermatologists who believe that coal tar is still the most effective sensitizing agent for the sun's radiation. More common for severe psoriasis, though, are oral medications that make a patient's skin highly sensitive to sunlight and carefully controlled exposure to UVA radiation at a dermatology clinic (a treatment called psoralen UVA photochemotherapy, or PUVA). Over the years, more than thirty skin diseases have been shown to respond positively to PUVA treatment. This treatment is very effective, but PUVA therapy is quite inconvenient for the patient, who has to visit the clinic two or three times a week. Also, when done too many times, PUVA causes non-melanoma skin cancer, melanomas, and cataracts. PUVA is now considered outdated by some.

Until very recently, treatment for psoriasis was based on the premise that the disease of psoriasis starts with a defective immune system. I don't believe this to be the case and stated my claim in an editorial in the journal *Experimental Dermatology*. My research shows that although the immune system is certainly involved, the problem begins with a defect in the skin cells themselves. This defect causes the skin cells to reproduce out of control. Only after the skin cells start overproducing does the autoimmune system sense there's something wrong and get involved, which only causes the problem to get worse. In other words, in psoriasis the autoimmune response is *secondary* to the initial problem in the skin cells.

Until recently, most treatments for psoriasis have been designed to suppress the autoimmune system. Not only does this not address the root cause of the problem—a defect in the skin cells that causes them to reproduce out of control—but it can also have serious side effects. Medications to suppress the autoimmune system such as cyclosporine, prednisone, and methotrexate can raise blood pressure, damage the kidneys and liver, and cause osteoporosis, and topical steroids thin the skin (sometimes permanently). Suppressing the body's autoimmune system may also open the door to infection and skin cancer.

The new "gold standard" for treating psoriasis is a therapy I developed. I discovered that by applying to the affected skin an ointment made from activated vitamin D, it was possible to dramatically reduce the symptoms of psoriasis. Calcipotriene therapy was a natural progression of the research I had begun as a graduate student when I discovered the active form of vitamin D that provides humans with so many health benefits. This treatment differs from previous ones: Instead of suppressing the autoimmune response to skin cell defects, it corrects the skin cell defects themselves. We make our own activated vitamin D in the lab here at BU Medical Center, and we are able to test it on patients. In the United States, it is commercially available in synthetic form as calcipotriene from the drug company Bristol

Myers-Squibb under the brand name Dovonex. Patients apply the ointment or cream twice a day for six to eight weeks, and the vast majority experience moderate to good results within a matter of weeks. Unlike other forms of treatment for psoriasis, calcipotriene has no serious side effects (mild skin irritation may occur in sensitive areas). Calcipotriene is sometimes used in conjunction with a variety of other oral and topical medications, as well as exposure to UVB radiation from the sun or a sunlamp.

Can sunlight alone be used to treat psoriasis? Sunlight is, after all, a main source of vitamin D, and people with psoriasis seem to fare better during the summer months when it's sunnier. If I see someone who has a mild case of psoriasis and he or she never gets any natural sunlight, I advise the individual to spend more time in the sun to find out whether this alone is enough to treat the symptoms. If this measure is successful, then I would advise that person to use an indoor tanning facility during the nonsunny months. If the condition does not improve, the individual should seek the services of a dermatologist experienced in treating psoriasis with calcipotriene.

Along with other researchers, my colleagues and I found that the skin has the enzymatic machinery to activate vitamin D, the substance that most effectively prevents unhealthy cell reproduction of the sort characteristic of psoriasis.

The Future of Vitamin D Treatment

Scientists have understood the relationship between sunlight and bone health for about a century. It's only very recently, however, that the connection between sunlight and cellular health has become clear. Cells and organs throughout the body—including immune cells, colon, prostate, breast, and skin cells—have the ability to make their own activated vitamin D and use it to promote health and inhibit the kind of abnormal cell growth characteristic of diseases such as cancer.

Currently at the vitamin D lab at Boston University Medical School, we are researching ways to treat existing cancers of the breast, colon, and prostate with activated vitamin D. We are also investigating whether preventing vitamin D deficiency will decrease the risk of many cancers. The preliminary data are promising and support my underlying hypothesis that sunlight contributes to our overall health. Already we have found that we can prevent the spread of colon cancer in laboratory animals if they have adequate levels of vitamin D. Our goal is to develop a new approach for preventing and treating some cancers. You'll be hearing more and more about these kinds of studies in the future.

What can *you* do to make the best use of your body's ability to make activated vitamin D? Disease prevention is in your hands. It is almost impossible to get enough vitamin D from diet. By getting the appropriate amount of sun exposure and thereby ensuring that you have healthy vitamin D levels in your body, you will be taking large strides toward reducing your risk of a variety of life-threatening diseases. Specific guidelines on how much sun you need to establish and maintain healthy levels of vitamin D are provided in chapter 7.

CHAPTER FIVE

Light Up Your Life

How sunlight affects your psychological health and sleep patterns

Y OU KNOW THAT lingering sensation you have after spending a day at the beach? You feel on top of the world— happy, content, and relaxed. Countless poets and songwriters have written in praise of sunshine and how it makes them feel. Knowing that sunrise strikes such a positive chord, advertisers frequently use images of people sipping their coffee while the sun comes up. "Sunshine in a bottle" is the refrain of one orange juice maker who capitalizes on our innate affection for the sun when marketing its product. The fact of the matter is that sunlight plain old makes people *feel better*—and everyone knows it.

There are good reasons sunlight improves your outlook on life. Sun exposure provides a natural high by stimulating the release of "feel good" substances in your body, such as serotonin, dopamine, and beta endorphins. Sunshine also suppresses hormones like melatonin, which make you feel sluggish and "down." No wonder people feel so good after spending time in the sun!

New evidence shows that the human body produces these feel good substances in response to sunlight in more ways than were previously understood. For example, until recently most scientists believed only the brain produced beta endorphin—a substance that makes you feel happy and revived. My colleagues and I have proven in our laboratory that the skin also produces beta endorphins in response to UVB exposure. These beta endorphins, in turn, may enter the bloodstream and travel to the brain. In an indoor tanning facility, if you are wearing eye protection that prevents light signals from reaching your brain to stimulate serotonin and suppress melatonin, you will still experience that pronounced sense of well-being—your skin has produced the beta endorphins that may make you feel so invigorated.

Sunshine has more than a short-term impact on your psychological state. It almost completely controls the biological tempo of your life—your daily pattern of body temperature highs and lows, levels of alertness, sleeping patterns, hormonal secretions, and other basic biological functions such as when you eat and sleep.

The cycle of changes you undergo every day is known as your circadian rhythm. But it is only in the past few years that scientists have begun to understand how this affects your ability to think and act. Indeed, until the early 1980s, scientists believed human beings had evolved to a point where we controlled our own circadian rhythms.

In fact, we now know that circadian rhythms are controlled by a "biological clock" that is kept on a twenty-four-hour schedule by sunlight. Without sunshine and darkness signals,

UV Radiation: It Does a Mood Good!

Have you ever used a tanning bed or any other kind of artificial tanning source that contains UVB radiation? If so, you are one of the tens of millions of Americans who understand the feeling of well-being after exposure to UVB radiation from the sun or a tanning bed that emits UVB. Many people—health professionals included—used to believe it was the warmth of the tanning device that made them feel better. We now know that this "warm and fuzzy" feeling you get after being exposed to UV radiation has a scientific basis. In response to UV radiation, your brain produces serotonin and your skin produces beta endorphins. Both of these "feel good" substances will improve your mood.

your sleep/wake schedule would shift forward by an hour every day—or "free run"—as it does in submariners, astronauts, and anyone else who lives without natural sunlight.

Your biological clock is made up of a small cluster of cells called the *suprachiasmatic nucleus* (SCN), which is located near the center of the brain. Sunlight hits the photoreceptors in the retina of your eye, and this signal travels via the optic nerve to the hypothalamus, your brain's emotional command center, where the SCN is located. In addition to housing the SCN, the hypothalamus is responsible for a variety of involuntary functions that control your mood. One of the most important jobs of the hypothalamus is to send signals to the pineal gland. When it is dark outside, the gland releases a substance called melatonin, which makes your system slow down and sends you to sleep. Conversely, when the SCN receives signals that it is

What About Vitamin D?

Spending more time in the sun to improve your circadian rhythm health may also improve your vitamin D status, but the bright light treatments that are at the heart of modern treatment of circadian rhythm disorders will not increase the vitamin D in your bloodstream. The light boxes used to administer these treatments filter out all UVB radiation. Conversely, indoor tanning facilities where you might improve your vitamin D status have not been proven to benefit circadian rhythm health because you need to shield your eyes to prevent eye inflammation and cataracts when using such equipment. Indoor tanning facilities do improve your mental state, however, possibly because of the beta endorphins created by the skin in response to UVB exposure.

sunny, it sends messages to the pineal gland to shut down production of melatonin and increase production of the chemical serotonin, which makes you feel happy and alert.

Why are we so powerfully affected by sunlight? When our ancestors were first evolving, there wasn't a heck of a lot to do after the sun set but find somewhere comfy to sleep and rest for the next day. Thus, our physiology evolved in such a way as to shut down when darkness began and start up in response to sunlight. It isn't just the wake-and-sleep cycle that is affected by your circadian rhythms—a variety of other psychological and physical functions are profoundly influenced as well.

You may not give much thought to your circadian rhythms. You probably take for granted that you will be sleepy at night and then awake and alert during the daytime. Your mood may vary, but you manage to navigate life's pools and eddies—and its occasional storms—while keeping an even keel. Some days you may wake up on the wrong side of the bed, but for the most part you are reasonably good-humored. Guess what? All of that has something to do with your circadian rhythms. If your circadian rhythms are synchronized with your daily life, then chances are your mood state will be a healthy one. However, millions of people have circadian rhythm dysfunction, and they experience mood-related problems such as seasonal affective disorder and other forms of depression, premenstrual tension, and sleeping disorders. Circadian rhythm disorders are also thought to be associated with *physical* illnesses, including heart disease and gastrointestinal disorders.

Based on our growing understanding of the importance of sunshine on the functioning of the biological clock, scientists are now able to successfully treat most mood-related circadian rhythm–related conditions using artificial bright light. The message from this is a familiar one: Natural sunlight is something to be revered as being as essential to human health and well-being as food, water, and exercise.

Seasonal Affective Disorder (SAD)

If you live at higher latitudes, you are probably aware of some minor changes in yourself that accompany the lengthening days. Because there's less light—in terms of both intensity and duration—your hibernation impulse makes you want to eat more and be less energetic. Most of us cope quite well with these changes, and indeed, some become energized by the prospect of brisk January days and winter sports.

However, a significant number of people are extremely sensitive to changes in the length of the day, so much so that for them living a normal life in the modern age is difficult. In winter, their biological clocks tell them to hibernate even though life tells them there is work to do, PTA meetings to attend, the nightly news to watch, and kids to feed. Most of these people find it difficult to fulfill the everyday demands of life during the winter months.

This syndrome has been known for millennia. Hippocrates identified it in the time of the ancient Greeks. On May 16, 1898, Arctic voyager Dr. Frederick Cook wrote poignantly of psychological changes his fellow explorers were experiencing in response to the lack of sunlight:

> The winter and the darkness have slowly but steadily settled over us. . . . It is not difficult to read on the faces of my companions their thoughts and moody dispositions. . . . The curtain of blackness which has fallen over the outer world of icy desolation has also descended upon the inner world of our souls. Around the tables . . . men are sitting about sad and dejected, lost in dreams of melancholy from which, now and then, one arouses with an empty attempt at enthusiasm. For brief moments some try to break the spell by jokes, told perhaps for the fiftieth time. Others grind out a cheerful philosophy, but all efforts to infuse bright hopes fail.

This condition was formally identified in 1984 by Dr. Norman Rosenthal of the National Institute for Mental Health and was given the name seasonal affective disorder, or SAD (a highly appropriate acronym). Rosenthal established that this was a bona fide disorder by taking a group of people who re-

Symptoms of SAD

The "blahs" or "cabin fever" are not the same as SAD. Symptoms of full-blown SAD include the following:

- Depression that begins in fall or winter
- Lack of energy
- Decreased interest in work or important activities
- Increased appetite with weight gain
- Carbohydrate and sugar cravings
- Increased need for sleep and excessive daytime sleepiness
- Social withdrawal
- Extreme afternoon slumps with decreased energy and concentration
- Decreased sex drive

ported serious symptoms of "winter depression" and tracking them through the various seasons. With startling accuracy, he showed how their symptoms worsened with the shortening days and improved as the days got longer. Since Rosenthal's landmark study, many other researchers have confirmed his findings.

How do you know if you have SAD? The characteristic symptom of SAD is the onset of major depressive feelings at certain times of the year. Physical activity decreases. You feel very lethargic and even sluggish. Almost any physical activity seems to be too much effort. On the other hand, your appetite increases and you have a particular craving for carbohydrates and sugars such as starches, pastries and other sweets, and alcohol. This explains why people with SAD usually put on weight during the winter. Most people with SAD sleep for long hours—or wish they could! They may lose interest in sex, become irritable and bad-tempered, and have trouble thinking clearly and quickly, which may lead to mistakes.

Epidemiologists estimate that 2 to 3 percent of Americans develop full-blown SAD, with another 7 percent suffering a less extreme form of this condition. Women are four times as likely to get SAD, and the average age of onset is twenty-three. Because winter days get shorter at higher latitudes, the farther you live from the equator, the greater the chance you'll develop SAD. About 1.5 percent of people who live in Florida get SAD, while this condition afflicts almost 10 percent of people in New Hampshire.

The term "Holiday Blues" has been used to describe SAD. That's because in the northern hemisphere, the onset of SAD symptoms begins when people are gearing up for Thanksgiving, Christmas, and the New Year, and the omnipresent good cheer contrasts with many people's "blue mood." Until Dr. Rosenthal published his study, many people thought the holiday season itself was responsible for arousing depressive feelings in those who couldn't be with their loved ones or who felt stress in anticipation of family get-togethers.

What exactly is happening to people who develop SAD? I described earlier how darkness causes the pineal gland to release melatonin to make us slow down and go to sleep. Winter wreaks havoc with some people's physiology, and unlike the rest of us, individuals with SAD aren't able to suppress the production of melatonin in their system.

SAD is a major depressive syndrome with clinical manifestations. Thanks to the pioneering work of doctors like Norman

Guidelines for Minimizing the "Winter Blahs"

If your spirits inevitably sink a little during the winter months, you may not have seasonal affective disorder but a less serious, or "subclinical," version of this condition colloquially referred to as the "winter blahs." Be attuned to your moods and energy levels. If you start feeling "low" toward the end of summer, take preventive action, including some of the following measures:

- Get as much natural sunlight as possible. When it's sunny, spend as much time as you can outdoors.
- If you are at home during the day, keep the curtains open as much as possible.
- If you work in an office, try to get a workspace that's near a window.
- Be physically active, and begin your physical activity *before* the symptoms start.
- Try to establish a mind-set that will enable you to enjoy the wintertime. You can't stop it coming, so gear up to get as much as you can out of it!
- Plan active events for yourself in advance of the fall. Schedule things to look forward to.

If you feel yourself succumbing, don't feel ashamed or try to hide it. You are by no means alone. Seek competent professional help. What you learn this winter you can apply to winter seasons to come.

Rosenthal, it is now listed in the American Psychiatric Association's standard text, the *Diagnostic and Statistical Manual of Mental Disorders*. In the past, SAD has been treated using strong antidepressant drugs and even electric shock therapy. However, by far the most effective treatment for SAD is sunlight, or artificial bright light that replicates the effect of sunshine. In

Norman Rosenthal's study, he told a large group of patients that he was going to expose them to bright light, which may or may not help their condition. He exposed half the patients to the kind of high intensity light that simulates midday sunshine (between 5,000 and 10,000 lux; a lux is a measurement of light) and the rest to the equivalent to bright indoor household light (bright office lighting emits between 500 and 700 lux, which is equal only to the light at dusk or dawn). The patients did not know which type of light therapy they were getting. Almost all the SAD patients who were exposed to the high-intensity lights experienced a dramatic reduction in symptoms, whereas those in the yellow light group saw no improvement. Numerous studies have duplicated these results.

Bright light treatment administered by a "light box" is now the treatment of choice if you have SAD. Eighty percent of people with SAD benefit from it. It's important to have a qualified doctor provide you with guidelines for using your light box, although you will find through trial and error what works best for you. (Refer to pages 142–145 for specifics on light boxes.)

Therapists usually have their SAD patients start with a single ten- to fifteen-minute session every day, gradually increasing their exposure to thirty to forty-five minutes. If your symptoms persist or worsen as the days lengthen, do two sessions a day. Total exposure should be limited to between ninety minutes and two hours. Studies have shown that morning bright light sessions work better at treating the symptoms of SAD.

The *Clinical Practice Guidelines* issued by the U.S. Department of Health and Human Services recognize bright light as a

The Importance of
Taking Depression Symptoms Seriously

Just because your depression symptoms occur only at certain times of the year doesn't mean they are all in your head. The symptoms of depression—seasonal or nonseasonal—must be taken very seriously. Proper diagnosis and treatment is essential. If you experience persistent sadness that lasts for more than two weeks, accompanied by problems with sleep, appetite, concentration, and energy, seek professional help. This is especially important if you are experiencing thoughts of suicide or of hurting yourself. If you can't immediately reach your primary care physician, many communities have telephone hotlines that offer immediate support. If there is no such service nearby, call the nearest emergency room or health care facility. Remember, there is a tried and tested way for you to feel better!

generally accepted treatment for SAD. However, on the rare occasion that bright light treatments don't work, antidepressant medications may be prescribed for use in conjunction with this kind of therapy.

Keep in mind that the light boxes used to treat SAD are *not* sunlamps, so you will not get a tan from them—nor any vitamin D benefits.

SAD symptoms usually improve after just a few days of bright light therapy. The best results are seen in people who stick to a consistent schedule beginning in the fall or winter and continuing until the spring. A common mistake is to discontinue treatments as soon as you feel better. In such cases, the symptoms return. This reinforces the need to keep up treatments throughout the winter months.

Nonseasonal Depression

There are different degrees of nonseasonal depression.

- Mild depression, the "blues," may be brought on by an unhappy event, such as a divorce or the death of a relative, and is characterized by feelings of sadness, gloominess, or emptiness, which may be accompanied by lethargy.

- Chronic low-grade depression, also known as *dysthymia*, exists when a person feels depressed most of the time for a period of two years. These feelings are accompanied by changes in energy, appetite, or sleep, as well as low self-esteem and feelings of hopelessness.

- Major depression involves severe, persistent mood depression and loss of interest and pleasure in daily activities, accompanied by decreased energy, changes in sleep and appetite, and feelings of guilt or hopelessness. These symptoms must be present for at least two weeks, cause significant distress, and be severe enough to interfere with functioning. If the depression is very severe, it may be accompanied by psychotic symptoms or by suicidal thoughts or behaviors.

Until recently, few studies had measured the effect of bright light on nonseasonal depression. The success of bright light treatment on seasonal affective disorder, however, has prompted numerous researchers to study whether this therapy would be effective for the treatment of nonseasonal depression. The results have been extremely encouraging.

Several studies have shown that bright light therapy alone is as effective as antidepressant medications in reducing the symptoms of nonseasonal depression. One study showed that just a single hour of bright light treatment was as effective as several weeks on a standard medication for depression. Some of the most significant work in this area is being done at the University of California at San Diego and at the University of Vienna in Austria. Researchers at these institutions have found that combining bright light therapy and antidepressant medications is an extremely successful way to alleviate the symptoms of depression.

Bright light therapy is a fundamental component of the latest and most successful treatment for nonseasonal depression. This form of therapy involves a triple-effect: bright light exposure, antidepressant medication, and "wake therapy." In wake therapy, patients wake themselves halfway through the night on the first night their program begins and stay awake until they have their bright light treatment at around breakfast time (these patients had already begun antidepressant medications, so the effects of the drug had begun). Wake therapy seems to intensify the effectiveness of the bright light therapy, perhaps because it jump-starts the suppression of melatonin production and increases serotonin production. Patients who have undergone this "triple-whammy" depression therapy have experienced a 27 percent decrease in symptoms in one week.

The success of bright light in treating depressive disorders has inspired doctors to use this therapy to treat conditions

How Researchers Measure Mood
Before and After Light Treatments

There's no mechanical device to measure depression, so how do doctors tell if antidepression treatments such as bright light are working?

Scientists rate how depressed patients are before and after treatment with "depression rating scales." They interview patients and ask them to score how sad, guilty, without appetite, suicidal, and so forth they are, and then add up the points to reach a total depression score. After therapy, the researchers ask the same questions. If the score is the same or higher, they conclude that the treatment made no difference or perhaps made the patient's condition worse. But if the score is lower, the treatment has worked.

ranging from bulimia, chronic fatigue syndrome, post- and antepartum depression, alcohol withdrawal syndrome, adolescent depression, jet lag, and certain forms of mental illness.

Premenstrual Syndrome (PMS)

Premenstrual syndrome (PMS) refers to a group of symptoms that occurs regularly in conjunction with a woman's monthly menstrual period. The symptoms tend to occur five to eleven days before her period starts and stop when her period begins.

Most women are affected by PMS at some point during their childbearing years. Between 30 and 40 percent of women have PMS symptoms severe enough to interfere with daily living, and 10 percent suffer symptoms so severe they are debilitating.

PMS is extremely trying for the woman who suffers from it, and it can cause extreme difficulties for her relationships with friends, family, and colleagues.

The incidence of PMS is higher in those between their late twenties and early forties, those with at least one child, those with a family history of a major depression disorder, or those with a past medical history of either postpartum depression or some other affective mood disorder, such as SAD.

It used to be thought that PMS symptoms were caused by a hormonal imbalance that occurred during the menstrual cycle. Now it's understood that PMS is a result of insufficient serotonin—a chemical that carries messages between the nerves and makes us feel calm, happy, and alert. Just before a woman gets her period, her levels of serotonin naturally drop and then go back up again when her period starts. If she has naturally low base levels of serotonin, symptoms of PMS will probably occur as serotonin levels drop below the point at which they are needed to maintain good psychological health.

Several researchers have demonstrated that PMS responds well to bright light treatment. The reason bright light works to reduce the symptoms of PMS is quite straightforward: Serotonin levels in the body increase in response to bright light. One of the most important recent studies of how bright light can be used to treat PMS was led by Dr. D. J. Anderson and published in the *Journal of Obstetrics and Gynaecology*. Dr. Anderson's six-month study involved a group of twenty women who had unsuccessfully tried in a variety of other ways to reduce their serious, ongoing problems with PMS. The women were exposed to fifteen to twenty-nine minutes of bright light therapy every day for four consecutive menstrual periods. At the end of the study,

Symptoms of Premenstrual Syndrome

You have PMS if five or more of these symptoms are associated with your menstrual period:

- Feeling of sadness or hopelessness, possible suicidal thoughts
- Feelings of tension or anxiety
- Mood swings marked by periods of teariness
- Persistent irritability or anger that affects other people
- Disinterest in daily activities and relationships
- Trouble concentrating
- Fatigue or low energy
- Food cravings or binging
- Sleep disturbances
- Feeling out of control
- Physical symptoms, such as bloating, breast tenderness, headaches, and joint or muscle pain

Dr. Anderson and his colleagues found that the bright light treatments had reduced by 76 percent the severity of PMS symptoms such as depression, anxiety, irritability, poor concentration, fatigue, food cravings, bloating, and breast pain.

If you have serious PMS, contact a physician and ask for a referral to a health care professional qualified to prescribe bright light treatments.

Shift Worker Syndrome

Tens of millions of Americans work the night shift. Night shift workers experience a variety of problems, such as a higher risk of psychological ailments and an increased like-lihood of fatigue-related accidents. Night workers also have higher rates of heart disease, cancer, diabetes, and gastro-intestinal disorders.

Despite the additional expense of paying people to work the night shift and the problems it causes for the workers, in this modern age we need people working unfavorable hours. Certain industries, such as oil refining, need to operate around the clock; others find it economically desirable to keep the as-sembly line moving; emergency response and law enforcement need personnel operating their stations twenty-four hours a day; and convenience stores need to keep their doors open in case someone needs a gallon of milk at two o'clock in the morning.

Night shift workers experience problems because their lives operate in opposition to their circadian rhythms. No matter how long a person works the night shift, when he leaves work and walks into the daylight to go home to bed, his body clock tells him it is time to wake up. That makes it hard for that per-son to get a full night's sleep during the day.

Studies of night shift workers have shown that, on average, they sleep one to two hours less than a day worker. That sleep loss is cumulative and is primarily responsible for the problems night shift workers tend to have staying alert during their shift and experiencing a fulfilling life outside of work.

A large number of studies have shown that bright light therapy is extremely helpful in helping night shift workers adapt to their work schedules. Companies that have employees working the night shift should fully utilize bright light technol-ogy to improve worker morale and reduce errors and accidents

Guidelines for Decreasing
Circadian Rhythm Disruptions Caused by Shift Work

- Reduce the number of consecutive night shifts you work. Night shift workers get less sleep than day workers. Over several days, they become progressively more sleep deprived. If you limit the number of third shifts you work to five or fewer, with days off in between, you are more likely to recover from sleep deprivation. If you work a twelve-hour shift instead of the usual eight hours, limit this to four consecutive shifts. After several consecutive night shifts, you should ideally receive a forty-eight-hour break.

- Avoid working prolonged shifts, working excessive overtime, and taking only short breaks.

- Avoid long commutes because they waste time you could spend sleeping.

- Avoid rotating shifts more than once a week. It is more difficult to cope with such alteration than it is to work the same shift for extended periods. The sequence of shift rotation can be important as well. Working the first shift, then the second shift, and then the third shift is easier than working the first, the third, and then the second shift.

- Get enough sleep on your days off. Practice good "sleep hygiene" by planning and arranging a sleep schedule and by avoiding caffeine, alcohol, and nicotine to help you sleep or stay awake.

- Avoid reliance on stimulants, over-the-counter and otherwise. Caffeine and stay-awake pills only temporarily trick the body into thinking it is functioning properly, which will only further disrupt your circadian rhythms.

on the job. The keys to this are having the appropriate bright light equipment installed and timing its use to synchronize workers' body clocks to the working and sleeping hours.

Elder Care

Bright light is being used with increasing frequency and success to treat a variety of disorders that affect our older citizens, especially sleep pattern disturbances and forms of dementia such as Alzheimer's disease.

Alzheimer's Disease

Alzheimer's disease is a progressive, degenerative disease of the brain that causes impaired memory, thinking, and behavior. People with Alzheimer's suffer disturbances in circadian rhythm because of the damage occurring to their brains. A vicious cycle often begins, with the Alzheimer's-induced circadian rhythm disturbances exacerbated by indoor confinement and lack of exercise, both of which contribute to circadian rhythm disorders.

A person with Alzheimer's typically has problems sleeping through the night. Night wanderings are common due to confusion and the inability to sleep. This can put an enormous strain on a caregiver, who may be an elderly spouse or a family member who has a full-time job to go to the next day.

Sedatives have traditionally been used to treat circadian rhythm symptoms associated with Alzheimer's, but they are not particularly effective and have significant side effects. A number of studies have proven that bright light treatments are extremely helpful for people with Alzheimer's. Bright light therapy helps people with Alzheimer's and other forms of dementia by resetting their biological clocks, helping them become more alert during the day so they go on fewer night wanderings. In addition, recent research has shown that reducing circadian rhythm disturbances using bright light treatments can improve the mental function of people with early-stage Alzheimer's disease. If you are caring for someone with Alzheimer's, do as much as you can to make sure that person is exposed to light during the early part of the day. To improve your charge's situation, get advice on bright light treatments from someone who has expertise in this area.

Sleep Disturbances

As people get older, their circadian rhythms "flatten out" and they become predisposed to sleep disturbances. This usually manifests itself in going to sleep too early and then waking before the sun comes up—often at three or four o'clock in the morning. In the most extreme cases, elderly nursing home patients may sleep at any hour of the day or night, sometimes even sleeping for part of every hour in the day.

Bright light therapy first thing in the morning following the same guidelines for seasonal affective disorder has been effective at resetting elderly people's biological clocks and restoring their circadian rhythms. Increasingly, attention is being paid to the kinds of lighting that should be provided for seniors, not just in the form of directed therapy but also as it should be

Sleep Tips

Want a better night's sleep? Try the following:

- Cut down on caffeine (including caffeinated soda) and avoid alcohol.
- Drink fewer fluids before going to sleep so you won't be awakened by bladder discomfort.
- Avoid heavy meals close to bedtime.
- Avoid nicotine.
- Exercise regularly, but do so in the early afternoon, not late afternoon or evening.
- Relax in a hot tub or bath before bedtime.
- Establish a regular bedtime and waketime schedule.

If your sleep problems become chronic, consider bright light therapy. Even people with mild sleeping disorders can benefit from bright light treatment. For example, a person who wants to go to sleep at eleven in the evening but can't nod off until one in the morning can reset the body's clock by having a leisurely breakfast in front of a light box.

incorporated into the design and architecture of homes and group living facilities.

Sleep Disorders

Millions of Americans suffer from sleep disorders—not being able to sleep enough, sleeping too much, or not being able to sleep at the right time. Frequently this is caused by a malfunction in the internal biological clock, which regulates sleep cycles. Under normal circumstances, a person's biological clock is set by the natural environment—especially the day and night.

Sleep disorders can occur when people's biological clocks get delayed or advanced from their natural environment. If you have *delayed* sleep phase syndrome, your clock is set *later*. You may find it difficult to fall asleep until the early hours of the morning—sometimes two or three o'clock—and may not be alert until noontime or later. People with *advanced* sleep phase syndrome have a biological clock that is set *earlier* than their natural environment. They tend to feel groggy and tired in the afternoon, fall asleep in the very early evening, then wake up in the middle of the night without being able to fall back to sleep.

Sleep disorders have been successfully treated with bright light therapy. The timing of the light treatments is key. People with delayed sleep phase syndrome can reset their biological clocks with early morning bright light treatments. Those who have advanced sleep phase syndrome will benefit from late afternoon or early evening bright light treatments.

All About Light Boxes

Light boxes emit up to 10,000 lux and replicate the intensity of natural sunshine at around noontime. The light emitted by these devices is twenty times the intensity of average indoor light (500 to 1,000 lux), which, most people are surprised to find out, is only as strong as the natural twilight. People with circadian rhythm disorders use light boxes to treat their individual conditions.

The light boxes themselves consist of a set of fluorescent bulbs installed in a box with a diffusing screen that spreads the light evenly and filters out all UVB and most UVA radiation. You position the box on a nearby table or desktop and sit comfortably for the treatment session. You will need to sit or stand close to the light box, with or without the room lights on, and your eyes must be open. You do not need to look at the lights; instead, use the time to read, write, watch TV, or eat a meal. The only reported side effects are occasional slight headaches.

The duration of bright light treatment sessions varies from fifteen minutes to three hours a day depending on your individual needs and the equipment you use. The more powerful the unit, the less time you have to spend in front of it to get the same effect. For example, to get the same benefit from a 10,000 lux light box as from a 2,500 lux light box, you need to spend only a quarter the amount of time in front of it—fifteen minutes instead of an hour, for example. Also, the nearer you are to the light source, the higher the intensity of light shining through your eyes, and the quicker and more effective the treatment.

Timing of light treatments is extremely important and varies with each person. Some people need two short treatments a day; others should have one long treatment in the morning or at night. This particularity reinforces the need to use bright light treatment under the supervision of a qualified sleep therapist.

Several reputable companies sell light boxes. Apollo Light Systems has been around longer than any other company in the field and has been recognized as the leader in light therapy for twenty years (for specific product information, visit their Web site at www.apollolight.com). Most innovations in home light therapy have originated with Apollo. The key to successful bright light treatment is a product that provides strong light at a reasonable unit-to-user distance, and Apollo sells products that do what they're advertised to do. Their popular Brite Lite IV unit puts out 10,000 lux from 28 inches away. They also make a unit that looks like a reading light that you can put on your office desk; this product projects 10,000 lux from 15 inches away. Apollo products also offer excellent service and durability.

It is important that you purchase your light box from a reputable company because there's no way you can measure the lux output of a bright light unit. If your symptoms don't improve, you wouldn't know if it was because the inexpensive light box you bought was not emitting strong enough light or because your condition was resistant to bright light treatment. Tests of products sold by disreputable companies demonstrate that certain light box units don't put out the amount of light they were advertised to. Also, poor quality screens may not filter out enough UV radiation and may damage your eyes.

Reputable companies will provide you with advice on which product you should buy. A portable unit might suit you if you travel a lot, or one with a stand may fit your needs if you plan to get bright light treatment while working out on a treadmill or stair climber. Numerous accessories are also available, including padded carrying cases and stands that let you place the light boxes in different positions. Reputable light box makers other than Apollo include Enviro Med (www.bio-light.com) and Northern Light Technologies (www.northernlight-tech.com). Distributors include Affordable Light Therapy (www .lighttherapy.com) and Amjo Corporation (www.sadlight.com).

Light boxes cost between $200 and $700, depending on a variety of factors, most important being their lux output and

---

Light Box Alternatives

Light boxes are the traditional way to undergo bright light therapy. Based on the success of this form of treatment for circadian rhythm disorders, alternatives to light boxes have been developed, including visors and goggles with lights built into them, which were pioneered by Dr. George Brainard. The obvious advantage of these products is that you don't have to stay still when using them.

---

the distance the unit can project that light intensity. Many insurance companies will reimburse the purchase price of light fixtures for the treatment of SAD, PMS, and sleep disorders. Reputable sellers can provide you with details.

You don't need a prescription for a light box, but anyone suffering from a serious mood-related disorder should certainly seek a doctor's recommendation before obtaining a unit and use it under the doctor's supervision. Choose your doctor wisely, and question one who only prescribes drugs such as sedatives or antidepressants for your condition. Some doctors are unaware of the successful results of bright light therapy.

The Future of Treatment for Circadian Rhythm Disorders

Bright light treatment is an exciting breakthrough in the treatment of mood-related conditions caused by circadian rhythm dysfunction. Treatments are safe and economical, and light boxes have no side effects. Light boxes represent a one-time cost of $200 to $700, versus $70 per month for an antidepressant such as Prozac. However, bright light treatments can be extremely effective when used in conjunction with antidepressant medications.

Recent breakthroughs have demonstrated that bright "blue light" treatments may have even more applications than we fully understand. For some time, blue light treatments have been used with great success for babies with jaundice. More recently, blue light treatments have been used to stimulate weight gain in premature babies.

New evidence from my laboratory—that it's not just our brains that make the powerful mood-enhancing beta endorphins in response to UVB exposure but our *skin* also—is another major step forward. Most recently, my colleagues and I identified two genes in the skin that are responsible for regulating the body's circadian rhythms.

Researchers have discovered that we have biological clocks all over our bodies, not just in the hypothalamus of our brains. These discoveries increase the likelihood that we may soon have the ability to treat a variety of other conditions associated with circadian rhythm disruption, including heart disease and diabetes.

CHAPTER SIX

When the Sun Just Isn't for You

Exploring other sources of vitamin D: Diet, supplements, and artificial sunlight

YOU NEED ENOUGH vitamin D in your bloodstream to ensure the health of your bones and to help prevent a variety of deadly diseases, including cancer, diabetes, and hypertension. How much vitamin D should you get every day? The government's recommendations are based on outdated science and are totally inadequate: 200 IU for children and adults up to age forty-nine, 400 IU for those ages fifty to seventy, and 600 IU for people overage seventy. As a vitamin D specialist, here is my recommendation: *All of us over age one need to get at least 1,000 IU of vitamin D every day.*

One of the reasons the government's recommendations are much lower than the levels that vitamin D specialists like me currently advocate is that when these guidelines were being formulated (and I was on the panel that was part of the process), we weren't able to consider information that at the time had yet to be proven but is now part of the scientific literature.

Our richest source of vitamin D is the sun. Most of us need only a few minutes a day of sun exposure during the summer months to maintain healthy vitamin D levels throughout the year. I have calculated that 25 to 50 percent of 1MED on your face, hands, and arms (or arms and legs) equals approximately 1,000 IU of vitamin D. (Remember that 1MED is the length of time in the sun at which your skin would typically begin to turn pink based on your previous experience.) If for some reason you can't get even that amount of sunlight—perhaps you work indoors or you simply can't work it into your schedule—then you have several options. Other than sunlight, the three principal sources of vitamin D are food and drink, supplements in pill form, and artificial sources of UVB radiation.

Vitamin D From Food and Drink

Eel, anyone? Care for a can of sardines? The modern American diet contains very little vitamin D. The kinds of foods rich in vitamin D tend to be very strong tasting and do not appeal to the American palate. It is really quite impractical to get 1,000 IU of vitamin D from diet alone because you would have to eat very large quantities of these vitamin D-rich foods.

The issue of vitamin D in milk is a contentious one. In response to the discovery in the 1920s that vitamin D was a cure for the childhood bone disease rickets, U.S. milk suppliers started putting vitamin D in milk in a variety of ways and marketing the milk as "vitamin D fortified." Initially this helped eradicate the scourge of rickets in American children. Many

Americans believe milk is their primary source of vitamin D and that even if they, as adults, don't drink enough of it, certainly their kids do.

An eight-ounce glass of vitamin D-fortified milk is supposed to contain 100 IU of vitamin D. However, a study my laboratory did revealed that most so-called vitamin D-fortified milk contains less than 20 percent of the amount listed on the label, half contains less than 50 percent, and 14 percent of the skim milk samples contain no detectable vitamin D. (This study has been backed by the research of other scientists.) We found that the vitamin D content even in the same brand of milk was arbitrary and varied from day to day. There is no way to tell when you're in the supermarket dairy section which milk contains the amount stated on its label. Finally, even if all milk *did* contain 100 IU of vitamin D, you would have to drink ten glasses of it every day to meet your vitamin D requirement!

A newer way of getting additional vitamin D in your diet is from orange juice and other juice products. Responding to the new information about the importance of vitamin D to health, Minute Maid now fortifies its premium chilled juices with as much vitamin D per serving as milk is supposed to have. I tested this product and found it not only contained the amount of vitamin D the manufacturer said it did but that it was also efficiently absorbed into the bloodstream.

The richest source of vitamin D is good old cod liver oil, which in its undiluted high-quality form contains a whopping 1,360 IU per tablespoon. If you are younger than forty years old, you may not have heard of cod liver oil, let alone tasted it. But for North Americans and northern Europeans, it was once the folk medicine of choice to prevent vitamin D deficiency.

Table 6.1 Holick Daily Value Estimates of the
Percentage of Vitamin D in Selected Foods

Food	IU	% HDV*
Salmon, cooked, 3½ oz	360	36
Mackerel, cooked, 3½ oz	345	35
Sardines, canned in oil, drained, 3½ oz	270	27
Eel, cooked, 3½ oz	200	20
Milk, nonfat, reduced fat, and whole, vitamin D fortified, 1 c (8 oz)	100	10
Margarine, fortified, 1 T	60	6
Cereal grain bars, fortified with 10 percent of the DV, 1 each	50	5
Pudding, ½ c prepared from mix and made with vitamin D fortified milk	50	5
Dry cereal, vitamin D fortified with 10 percent of DV, ¾ c (other cereals may be fortified with more or less vitamin D)	40–50	1
Liver, beef, cooked, 3½ oz	30	3
Egg, 1 whole (vitamin D is present in the yolk)	25	2.5

*HDV = Holick Daily Value

Generations of grim-faced parents administered spoonfuls of this slippery, slimy, fish-tasting liquid to their protesting offspring. Its impact was dramatic: It cured rickets in children who had this condition and prevented it in those at risk. Though it has gone out of fashion, cod liver oil continues to be an excellent vitamin D supplement. The good news is that cod liver oil is now available in a less disagreeable capsule form, which makes it much easier to consume (and administer to kids!).

My research and the research of others has demonstrated that we need 1,000 IU of vitamin D every day. Table 6.1 reflects *my* estimate of how much of your daily vitamin D intake a serving from each of these foods will provide based on a 2,000 calorie diet. Values may be higher or lower depending on your calorie needs.

Vitamin D Supplements

"Why don't I just take a supplement?" That's the attitude of many people when they hear the new findings about the benefits of vitamin D. Their rationale is that by taking a vitamin D supplement, they can avoid the health risks of sun exposure while still availing themselves of all the health benefits of this vitamin. Unfortunately, it's not that straightforward.

Few 1,000 IU vitamin D supplements are available. Solgar (www.solgar.com) is one reputable brand. Multivitamins contain 400 IU of vitamin D, so to get the amount of vitamin D you need from supplements alone, you would have to take two and a half multivitamins a day. This is impractical as well as expensive and potentially dangerous. More important, taking two and a half multivitamins will overload your body with vitamin A, which in excessive amounts has been associated with birth defects and osteoporosis.

If you overuse vitamin D supplements, you are at risk of vitamin D "toxicity," which you cannot develop by spending too much time in the sun or on a tanning bed. This condition involves a number of serious problems, including nausea,

Why Relaxing in the Sunshine
Beats Eating Mackerel and Popping Pills

Vitamin D in oral form—whether in whole foods or pill supplements—may not provide as many benefits as the vitamin D you get from the sun.

To begin with, the vitamin D you get from sunlight stays in your body for a longer time and therefore provides longer-lasting benefits. In addition, sunlight causes your body to make not just vitamin D itself but also beneficial vitamin D–related substances called *photoisomers*. We are currently doing research in this area at the Boston University Medical School.

Keep in mind that neither vitamin D–rich foods nor supplements will cause your body to produce feel-good substances such as beta endorphins and serotonin, which create the sense of well-being you feel after being in the sun or using an indoor tanning facility.

Finally, unlike vitamin D supplements, neither sun exposure nor a tanning bed can cause vitamin D toxicity.

vomiting, loss of appetite, constipation, and weight loss. Elevated calcium levels brought on by this condition can cause a variety of physical conditions, such as calcification of the kidneys causing kidney failure, calcification of the major arteries, and confusion and bizarre behavior. Vitamin D toxicity was what prompted European governments to ban vitamin D fortification of milk in the 1950s. At that time, European milk producers put too much vitamin D in their milk, and the health consequences in children caused public outrage. To avoid vitamin D toxicity, children over one year of age and adults should not take any more than 2,000 IU of vitamin D per day in oral form except under a doctor's supervision.

Although sunlight should be most people's main source of vitamin D, vitamin D supplements may be appropriate for persons taking certain antibiotics or antihypertension medications that make them sun sensitive. Supplements may also be useful for people with Type 1 or Type 2 skin who have trouble going out into the sun without getting burned. Always remember that supplements are no remedy for poor nutritional habits, so it's important to eat a well-balanced diet. Otherwise, a nutritional supplement will be ineffective.

If you live in a high latitude and spend plenty of time outside during the summer months, then taking a multivitamin during the winter may not be necessary, but it will make absolutely sure you have healthy vitamin D levels year round. To find out if you have enough vitamin D, you can get your status checked with a blood test (the doctor checks your 25-vitamin D levels, not your levels of activated vitamin D). This is done in a clinical setting. The doctor draws a small amount of your blood that is then sent to the lab for testing. Your 25-vitamin D levels should be no less than 20 nanograms per milliliter of blood (ng/ml) and should ideally be in the 30 to 50 ng/ml range.

Indoor Tanning Facilities

In a perfect world, all of us would have the time and opportunity to strip off our clothes and step outside for several minutes a day for the amount of sun we need to make enough vitamin D to be healthy. Regrettably, that's not the case, and real life (not to mention office dress codes) tends to interfere with this goal.

Every day, approximately one million Americans frequent an indoor tanning facility to look and feel better. Although I am not an advocate of tanning per se, I do believe in the importance of UVB exposure for making the vitamin D you need to be healthy and feel invigorated. If you don't have the opportunity to go out in the sun or prefer a more private and controlled environment, indoor tanning facilities represent a viable alternative to natural sunshine.

I also am a realist and believe many of you will continue to frequent indoor tanning facilities because of the way you look and feel afterward. I also believe if you have all the facts, you have the right to make the choice to enjoy UVB exposure. With all this in mind, if you choose to tan indoors, make sure you use this technology *responsibly*.

Thankfully, the indoor tanning industry, through the efforts of the Indoor Tanning Association, is doing its part by introducing quality control measures and offering education and certification for its personnel.

Keep in mind that there's no such thing as artificial UV radiation. A UVB photon packet of energy is a photon no matter how it is produced. Artificial *sources* of energy do exist, and among these sources are the lamps used in indoor tanning facilities.

The fact that the radiation you are exposed to in indoor tanning facilities is the same as what you get from the sun means you need to take the same precautions you would if you were in the natural sunlight. As with natural sunlight, when using indoor tanning equipment, there is the potential for the kind of overexposure that is associated with skin cancer and prematurely aged skin.

Above all, make sure the indoor tanning facility you use features appropriate equipment. At one time, indoor tanning facilities used equipment that emitted high-intensity UVB radiation. When UVB radiation was linked to basal cell and squamous cell skin cancer, the industry switched to UVA-only "high-pressure" lamps, which were considered safe because they didn't cause burning. Then it was discovered that UVA radiation may contribute to melanoma and wrinkles as well as increase the risk of non-melanoma skin cancer. Therefore, the trend in recent times has been toward low-pressure lamps that emit a balance of UVA and UVB radiation (94%–97.5% UVA to 2.5%–6% UVB) that replicates natural sunshine. Before using an indoor tanning facility, make sure it features low-pressure lamps. Facilities that use high-pressure lamps should be avoided not only because of the potential of those lamps for causing skin damage and certain types of cancers, but also because they do not provide any sort of vitamin D benefit.

If you require assistance, find a facility where the staff has been certified by an industry association such as the International Smart Tan Network. A qualified staff member should do the following:

- Discuss your skin type and exposure time charts carefully with you and ensure that you have access to this information at all times.

- Recommend an exposure schedule that will tan you moderately and avoid any pinkness, and especially sunburn.

- Discuss anything that may react adversely to UV exposure (certain medicines, birth control pills, cosmetics, or soaps may increase your risk of a sun-sensitive reaction).

- Provide you with FDA-approved eyewear with instructions on usage.

- Guide you through your first tanning experience.

Follow staff guidelines and those of the equipment manufacturers. Do not exceed the recommended exposure time. In fact, consider spending *less* time than is recommended. Indoor tanning exposure times are based on FDA and Federal Trade Commission guidelines, which allow a per-session UV exposure equivalent to 75 percent of 1MED. This is quite liberal because you require only 25 to 50 percent of 1MED (the time it would take you to get "pink") to get enough vitamin D (equivalent to taking about 4,000 to 10,000 IU of vitamin D orally).

If you are concerned about the potential harm of UVB radiation and are not interested in a tan, you can get all the medical benefits of UVB exposure from just 25 percent of 1MED (about 4,000 IU of vitamin D).

One of the most popular reasons for using indoor tanning facilities is to build a "base tan" in anticipation of a winter visit to a tropical destination such as the Caribbean. As I've made clear, I'm not a proponent of tanning, but I do believe in the importance of skin health and protecting it against strong sunshine. Increasing the melanin content in your skin by going to an indoor tanning facility will provide you with a certain amount of natural protection against a burn. Start increasing the melanin content in your skin by visiting an indoor tanning facility at least one month before you leave, and have three sessions a week. When you arrive at your tropical or subtropical destination, take the appropriate measures to protect yourself against a burn. Depending on your skin type, the protection

Guidelines for Indoor Tanning

- **Educate yourself.** Know the pros and cons of UV exposure and how to use and protect yourself.
- **Use low-pressure lamps.** Ask the attendant working at the facility whether he or she knows *for sure* that the lamps at that facility are low pressure (those that emit a balance of UVA and UVB). High-pressure lamps emit only UVA, which penetrates deep into the skin and may cause skin cancer and wrinkles.
- **Use common sense and practice moderation.** Refer to the guidelines in chapter 7 for how much UV exposure you need. Keep in mind that indoor tanning facilities emit UV radiation equivalent to the sunshine at mid-latitudes. Restrict your exposure to one-third to two-thirds of the maximum recommended exposure time.
- **Know the consequences of using oil.** Rubbing oil into your skin flattens the very top layer of skin (the stratum corneum) and increases the penetration of much of the UVA and UVB radiation that would otherwise be reflected off the skin. If you use such products, cut your UV exposure time in half.
- **Wear goggles or peepers.** Make sure the facility provides eyewear that fit snugly. If the facility offers goggles, make sure the goggles are sterilized after each use to prevent the spread of eye infections. If not, purchase your own pair of goggles.
- **Consider your medical history.** If you are being treated for lupus or tend to get cold sores, these conditions can be worsened through exposure to UV radiation from indoor tanning lamps, just as they are by natural sunlight. Your skin may also be more sensitive to UV radiation if you take certain medications such as antibiotics, antihistamines, tranquilizers, water pills, diuretics, or birth control pills. A well-run indoor tanning facility will keep a file with information about your medical history, medications, and treatments. Make sure you help the staff keep the file up to date.

you get from pre-vacation tanning salon exposure is equivalent to using a sunscreen with a sun protection factor of two or three (SPF2 or SPF3), which means you can stay outside two or three times longer than you could if you weren't wearing any sunscreen. Some people choose to purchase tanning equipment for use in their homes. I am in favor of doing this if your primary goal is to make vitamin D and improve your psychological health. Follow the same guidelines and precautions you would observe in commercial facilities or in natural sunshine. It is especially important to avoid overexposure, which can be a temptation because of your easy access to the equipment. Again, be sure your equipment uses low-pressure lamps—those that emit a balance of UVA and UVB radiation that most closely replicates natural sunlight.

Most people use tanning facilities for cosmetic reasons—in other words, to look and feel better. I use this kind of equipment extensively to test the effects of UV radiation on health. In one of the most dramatic examples of how indoor tanning equipment can be used therapeutically, I managed to relieve excruciating bone pain in a woman with severe Crohn's disease who was vitamin D deficient because 90 percent of her intestines had been removed in surgery and no amount of oral or intravenous vitamin D could enable her intestines to make enough vitamin D to keep her bones healthy. Her bone pain, caused by the condition known as osteomalacia (see chapter 4), was relieved in a month thanks to three-times-weekly sessions on a tanning bed observing manufacturer's exposure guidelines. If you have trouble absorbing vitamin D from your diet, speak to your doctor about whether indoor tanning sessions would help correct your vitamin D deficiency. Two of the most common conditions associated with difficulty absorbing vitamin D through the small intestine are Crohn's disease and cystic fibrosis.

Lamps that emit UVB radiation were originally invented to treat medical conditions in the 1940s. It was only later, when doctors discovered that their research subjects were also getting tanned, that an industry was born to take advantage of people's desire to look as if they had just returned from an expensive vacation in the tropics. With the new information that vitamin D is so important for good health, I hope you will start to regard indoor tanning facilities as places not to bronze yourself but rather to undergo therapy to stimulate your production of vitamin D.

CHAPTER SEVEN

R~X~: Sun

*Learning to use sunshine
as good medicine in everyday life*

THE MESSAGE I WANT TO SPREAD is that sunlight is as natural for human health as are food, water, oxygen, and physical activity. Healthy, moderate sun exposure establishes and maintains appropriate 25-vitamin D levels in your blood and may help prevent a variety of diseases, including cancer, stroke, heart attack, high blood pressure/hypertension, and autoimmune-related conditions such as Type 1 diabetes and multiple sclerosis. However, just because "some is good" doesn't mean that "a lot is better." Undesirable consequences can result if you get too much sun, just as if you eat or exercise too much. These consequences may include non-melanoma skin cancer, melanoma, and wrinkles.

If sun is essential for good health but too much can be unhealthy, this begs the obvious question: What is the right amount? I have been at the forefront of developing a scientific answer to this question and providing easy-to-use guidelines for the public.

I have calculated that to make approximately 800 to 1,500 IU of vitamin D you need to expose your face, hands, and arms or arms and legs (about 25 percent of your body) to between 25 and 50 percent of 1MED (1MED is when your skin gets pink from the sun). This calculation is based on my finding that exposure of 100 percent of your skin to 1MED will cause an increase in vitamin D in your body equivalent to taking between 10,000 and 25,000 IU of vitamin D orally. Again, I want to stress that I am not advocating that you actually get 1MED; you need to *estimate* this based on your skin type in order to calculate your safe and healthful sun exposure time.

I have developed two ways for you to get the right amount of sun exposure for good vitamin D health. One is a common-sense guideline that depends on knowing your tolerance for the sun (the Holick Formula for Safe Sun). The other relies on the wealth of available scientific data I have accumulated and incorporated into a specific user-friendly series of tables (the Holick Safe Sun Tables, see pages 166–177).

Sunscreens almost completely prevent the body from making any vitamin D from the sun. SPF8 reduces vitamin D production by 97.5 percent, and SPF15 reduces vitamin D production by 99.5 percent. Therefore, do not use any sunscreen during the time specified for safe sun exposure, but do put on a broad-spectrum sunscreen after that time has expired. Use a sunscreen with a sun protection factor of at least 15 so you can enjoy being outside without incurring any of the potentially harmful effects.

UVB radiation from sunlight does not penetrate glass, so you cannot make vitamin D from sunshine that warms your skin through a window.

I do not advocate tanning, and I recommend you get enough sun exposure only to establish and maintain healthy vitamin D levels and to improve your psychological health. At the same time, if you have decided that the feeling of well-being you get from UVB exposure far outweighs the dangers, I would not discourage you from UVB exposure in excess of that needed for good health, as long as you know and accept the risks. Spending time in the sun or using a tanning bed is an excellent way to ensure you will have healthy levels of vitamin D for optimal bone and cell health (remember that UVA tanning beds won't provide this benefit; you need to use ones with UVB in them).

In the interests of full disclosure, I tan responsibly by getting 25 to 50 percent of 1MED whenever the sun is strong enough to provide vitamin D benefit.

The Holick Formula for Safe Sun

I will describe here the Holick Formula for Safe Sun—my commonsense guideline for people who want to take advantage of the health benefits of sun exposure.

Here's how to use the Holick Formula to get safe amounts of sun exposure and make enough vitamin D for good health: Estimate how long it takes in the particular conditions you will be sunning yourself for you to get a mild sunburn (known as one minimal erythemal dose, or 1MED). Then, without applying

---

Holick Formula for Safe Sun

Expose 25 percent of your body's surface area to 25 percent of 1MED two to three times per week at all times of the year when you can make vitamin D in your skin (refer to tables—see page 166).

---

sunscreen, expose your hands, arms, and face for 25 percent of that length of time (or your arms and legs if you want to minimize facial wrinkling). I have calculated that that amount of sun exposure two to three days a week enables the body to make enough vitamin D to keep healthy. After getting this amount of sun exposure, you should put on sunscreen to lessen the risk of skin cancer and wrinkles. The more skin you expose to the sun, the more vitamin D you will make. If you are wearing a swimsuit, it will take you less time per session than 25 percent of 1MED to make the minimum amount of vitamin D you need for good health. Remember, it doesn't matter which area of your body is exposed to the sun so long as at least 25 percent is.

Here's an example of the Holick Formula in action. Say you live in New York and frequent the beaches of Long Island. If you have quite fair skin (Type 2 skin) and estimate it would take you half an hour to get "pink" on the beach at noontime in July because you haven't spent much time in the sun this summer season, then you should spend three to six minutes in the sun before putting on sunscreen. If you are wearing a bathing suit and are exposing 75 percent of your body to sunlight, then your time without a sunscreen can be reduced threefold to just one or two minutes.

What About Other Sources of Vitamin D?

Sunlight isn't the only source of vitamin D. In addition to a few vitamin D-rich foods, you can also get vitamin D from nutritional supplements and artificial sources of UVB radiation. These alternate sources are explained in chapter 6.

If you are a dark-skinned African American and can spend hours and hours out in the sun on the beaches of Long Island before getting burned—if you get burned at all—then spend half an hour in the sun before putting on any sunscreen. For those in between these two skin types who get pink in one hour, fifteen minutes of sun exposure will suffice.

You don't need to spend time on the beach to make vitamin D. You can do it sitting outside or walking while on your lunch break from work. But you do need to have your skin exposed to direct sunlight.

You cannot make vitamin D in high latitudes during the winter months. However, if you live in the northeastern United States and follow this guideline between May and October, you will make enough vitamin D to last you through the winter. Vitamin D is stored in your body fat and released in the winter when you need it. (However, if you are obese, this process is much less efficient, as the body tenaciously holds onto the vitamin D.) If you don't get this amount of sunlight between May and October, then during the winter months consider alternate forms of vitamin D, such as pill supplements and indoor tanning facilities (for guidelines on this, refer to chapter 6).

What if you live in a climate such as Florida where the sun shines all year round? The same principle applies. You should try to get a few minutes of sun exposure two to three times a week for a length of time that depends on your skin type.

Holick Safe Sun Tables

The second accurate and convenient method you can use to determine how much sun you need is with tables I have created based on my research. These tables provide safe sun time for different climactic locations and different skin types.

The most important things you need to know before you start is what skin type you have and what latitude category you are in. Pick your skin type from the following list, or to refresh your memory, refer to "What Skin Type Am I?" on page 39.

Type 1: fair-skinned; always burn and never tan

Type 2: burn easily and hardly tan

Type 3: sometimes burn and gradually tan

Type 4: rarely burn and always tan

Type 5: medium- to dark-skinned; seldom burn and always tan

Type 6: blue-black skin; never burn and tan darkly

For the tables I created, I divided the world into four main climactic regions: tropical, subtropical, mid-latitude, and high latitude. Refer to the map of the world (figure 7.1) or to the U.S. map (figure 7.2) to determine the region where you live or the regions where you will be getting sun exposure.

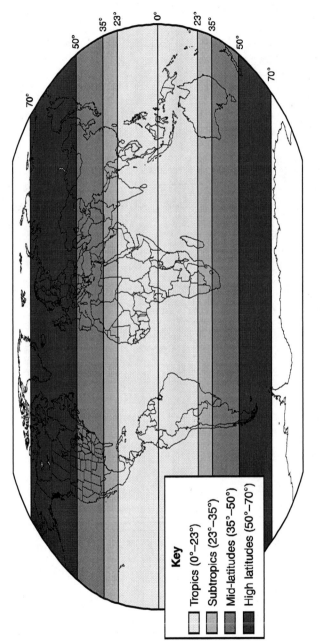

Figure 7.1 Map of the world

Key

Tropics (0°–23°)

Subtropics (23°–35°)

Mid-latitudes (35°–50°)

High latitudes (50°–70°)

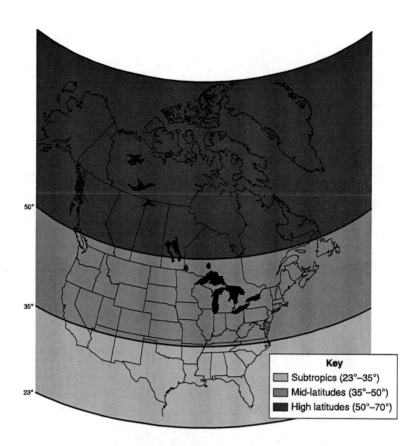

Figure 7.2 Map of North America

You can also use tables 7.1 and 7.2 to help you determine the region where you live and how much sun exposure is safe for you based on your skin type and the region and time of year.

Table 7.1. Latitude and Latitudinal Regions of U.S. and Canadian Cities

City	Latitude	Region	City	Latitude	Region
Albany, NY	42	Mid-latitudes	Carlsbad, NM	32	Subtropics
Albuquerque, NM	35	Subtropics	Charleston, SC	32	Subtropics
Amarillo, TX	35	Subtropics	Charleston, WV	38	Mid-latitudes
Anchorage, AK	61	High latitudes	Charlotte, NC	35	Subtropics
Atlanta, GA	33	Subtropics	Cheyenne, WY	41	Mid-latitudes
Austin, TX	30	Subtropics	Chicago, IL	41	Mid-latitudes
Baker, OR	44	Mid-latitudes	Cincinnati, OH	39	Mid-latitudes
Baltimore, MD	39	Mid-latitudes	Cleveland, OH	41	Mid-latitudes
Bangor, ME	44	Mid-latitudes	Columbia, SC	34	Subtropics
Birmingham, AL	33	Subtropics	Columbus, OH	40	Mid-latitudes
Bismarck, ND	46	Mid-latitudes	Dallas, TX	32	Subtropics
Boise, ID	43	Mid-latitudes	Denver, CO	39	Mid-latitudes
Boston, MA	42	Mid-latitudes	Des Moines, IA	41	Mid-latitudes
Buffalo, NY	42	Mid-latitudes	Detroit, MI	42	Mid-latitudes
Calgary, Alberta (CAN)	51	High latitudes	Dubuque, IA	42	Mid-latitudes

(continues)

Table 7.1. Latitude and Latitudinal Regions of U.S. and Canadian Cities *(continued)*

City	Latitude	Region	City	Latitude	Region
Duluth, MN	46	Mid-latitudes	Houston, TX	29	Subtropics
Eastport, ME	44	Mid-latitudes	Idaho Falls, ID	43	Mid-latitudes
El Centro, CA	32	Subtropics	Indianapolis, IN	39	Mid-latitudes
El Paso, TX	31	Subtropics	Jackson, MS	32	Subtropics
Eugene, OR	44	Mid-latitudes	Jacksonville, FL	30	Subtropics
Fargo, ND	46	Mid-latitudes	Juneau, AK	58	High latitudes
Flagstaff, AZ	35	Subtropics	Kansas City, MO	39	Mid-latitudes
Fort Worth, TX	32	Subtropics	Key West, FL	24	Subtropics
Fresno, CA	36	Mid-latitudes	Kingston, Ontario (CAN)	44	Mid-latitudes
Grand Junction, CO	39	Mid-latitudes	Klamath Falls, OR	42	Mid-latitudes
Grand Rapids, MI	42	Mid-latitudes	Knoxville, TN	35	Subtropics
Havre, MT	48	Mid-latitudes	Las Vegas, NV	36	Mid-latitudes
Helena, MT	46	Mid-latitudes	Lewiston, ID	46	Mid-latitudes
Honolulu, HI	21	Tropics	Lincoln, NE	40	Mid-latitudes
Hot Springs, AR	34	Subtropics	London, Ontario (CAN)	43	Mid-latitudes

Table 7.1. Latitude and Latitudinal Regions of U.S. and Canadian Cities *(continued)*

City	Latitude	Region	City	Latitude	Region
Los Angeles, CA	34	Subtropics	Nelson, British Columbia (CAN)	49	Mid-latitudes
Louisville, KY	38	Mid-latitudes	Newark, NJ	40	Mid-latitudes
Manchester, NH	43	Mid-latitudes	New Haven, CT	41	Mid-latitudes
Memphis, TN	35	Subtropics	New Orleans, LA	29	Subtropics
Miami, FL	25	Subtropics	New York, NY	40	Mid-latitudes
Milwaukee, WI	43	Mid-latitudes	Nome, AK	64	High latitudes
Minneapolis, MN	44	Mid-latitudes	Oakland, CA	37	Mid-latitudes
Mobile, AL	30	Subtropics	Oklahoma City, OK	35	Subtropics
Montgomery, AL	32	Subtropics	Omaha, NE	41	Mid-latitudes
Montpelier, VT	44	Mid-latitudes	Ottawa, Ontario (CAN)	45	Mid-latitudes
Montreal, Quebec (CAN)	45	Mid-latitudes	Philadelphia, PA	39	Mid-latitudes
Moose Jaw, Saskatchewan (CAN)	50	Mid-latitudes	Phoenix, AZ	33	Subtropics
Nashville, TN	36	Mid-latitudes	Pierre, SD	44	Mid-latitudes
			Pittsburgh, PA	40	Mid-latitudes

(continues)

Table 7.1. Latitude and Latitudinal Regions of U.S. and Canadian Cities *(continued)*

City	Latitude	Region	City	Latitude	Region
Port Arthur, Ontario (CAN)	48	Mid-latitudes	San Antonio, TX	29	Subtropics
Portland, ME	43	Mid-latitudes	San Diego, CA	32	Subtropics
Portland, OR	45	Mid-latitudes	San Francisco, CA	37	Mid-latitudes
Providence, RI	41	Mid-latitudes	San Jose, CA	37	Mid-latitudes
Quebec, Quebec (CAN)	46	Mid-latitudes	San Juan, Puerto Rico	18	Tropics
Raleigh, NC	35	Subtropics	Santa Fe, NM	35	Subtropics
Reno, NV	39	Mid-latitudes	Savannah, GA	32	Subtropics
Richfield, UT	38	Mid-latitudes	Seattle, WA	47	Mid-latitudes
Richmond, VA	37	Mid-latitudes	Shreveport, LA	32	Subtropics
Roanoke, VA	37	Mid-latitudes	Sioux Falls, SD	43	Mid-latitudes
Sacramento, CA	38	Mid-latitudes	Sitka, AK	57	High latitudes
St. John, New Brunswick (CAN)	45	Mid-latitudes	Spokane, WA	47	Mid-latitudes
St. Louis, MO	38	Mid-latitudes	Springfield, IL	39	Mid-latitudes
Salt Lake City, UT	40	Mid-latitudes	Springfield, MA	42	Mid-latitudes
			Springfield, MO	37	Mid-latitudes

Table 7.1. Latitude and Latitudinal Regions of U.S. and Canadian Cities (*continued*)

City	Latitude	Region	City	Latitude	Region
Syracuse, NY	43	Mid-latitudes	Virginia Beach, VA	36	Mid-latitudes
Tampa, FL	27	Subtropics	Washington, DC	38	Mid-latitudes
Toledo, OH	41	Mid-latitudes	Wichita, KS	37	Mid-latitudes
Toronto, Ontario (CAN)	43	Mid-latitudes	Wilmington, NC	34	Subtropics
Tulsa, OK	36	Mid-latitudes	Winnipeg, Manitoba (CAN)	49	Mid-latitudes
Victoria, British Columbia (CAN)	48	Mid-latitudes			

Table 7.2. Safe and Effective Sun Exposure for Vitamin D Production

Tropical Latitudes (approx. 0–23 degrees; Honolulu, Jamaica, U.S. Virgin Islands)

Time of Day	8 A.M.–11 A.M.				11 A.M.–3 P.M.				3 P.M.–6 P.M.			
Time of Year	Nov–Feb	Mar–May	Jun–Aug	Sep–Oct	Nov–Feb	Mar–May	Jun–Aug	Sep–Oct	Nov–Feb	Mar–May	Jun–Aug	Sep–Oct
Minutes of Sun												
Type 1 skin	10–15	5–10	3–5	5–10	5–10	3–8	1–5	3–8	10–15	5–10	3–5	5–10
Type 2 skin	15–20	10–15	5–10	10–15	10–15	5–10	2–8	5–10	15–20	10–15	5–10	10–15
Type 3 skin	20–30	15–20	10–15	15–20	15–20	10–15	5–10	10–15	20–30	15–20	10–15	15–20
Type 4 skin	30–45	20–30	15–20	20–30	20–30	15–20	10–15	15–20	30–45	20–30	15–20	20–30
Type 5–6 skin	45–60	30–45	20–30	30–45	30–45	20–30	15–20	20–30	45–60	30–45	20–30	30–45

Table 7.2. Safe and Effective Sun Exposure for Vitamin D Production *(continued)*

Subtropical Latitudes (approx 23–35 degrees; Miami, San Diego, Los Angeles)

Time of Day	8 A.M.–11 A.M.				11 A.M.–3 P.M.				3 P.M.–6 P.M.			
Time of Year	Nov–Feb	Mar–May	Jun–Aug	Sep–Oct	Nov–Feb	Mar–May	Jun–Aug	Sep–Oct	Nov–Feb	Mar–May	Jun–Aug	Sep–Oct
Minutes of Sun												
Type 1 skin	15–20	10–15	5–10	10–15	10–15	5–10	1–5	5–10	15–20	10–15	5–10	10–15
Type 2 skin	20–40	15–20	10–15	15–20	15–30	10–20	5–10	10–20	20–40	15–20	10–15	15–20
Type 3 skin	30–60	15–30	10–20	15–30	20–30	15–25	10–15	15–25	30–60	15–30	10–20	15–30
Type 4 skin	45–75	30–45	15–30	30–45	30–45	20–30	15–20	20–30	45–75	30–45	15–30	30–45
Type 5-6 skin	60–90	45–60	30–45	45–60	40–60	30–40	20–30	30–40	60–90	45–60	30–45	45–60

(continues)

Table 7.2. Safe and Effective Sun Exposure for Vitamin D Production (*continued*)

Mid–Latitudes (approx. 35–50 degrees; Hyannis, New York, San Francisco)

Time of Day	8 A.M.–11 A.M.				11 A.M.–3 P.M.				3 P.M.–6 P.M.			
Time of Year	Nov–Feb	Mar–May	Jun–Aug	Sep–Oct	Nov–Feb	Mar–May	Jun–Aug	Sep–Oct	Nov–Feb	Mar–May	Jun–Aug	Sep–Oct
Minutes of Sun												
Type 1 skin	0	15–20	10–15	15–20	0	10–15	2–8	10–15	0	15–20	10–15	15–20
Type 2 skin	0	20–30	15–20	20–30	0	15–20	5–10	15–20	0	20–30	15–20	20–30
Type 3 skin	0	30–40	20–30	30–40	0	30–40	15–20	30–40	0	30–40	20–30	30–40
Type 4 skin	0	40–60	30–40	40–60	0	30–40	20–25	30–40	0	40–60	30–40	40–60
Type 5–6 skin	0	60–75	40–60	60–75	0	40–60	25–35	40–60	0	60–75	40–60	60–75

Table 7.2. Safe and Effective Sun Exposure for Vitamin D Production (*continued*)

High Latitudes (approx. 50–75 degrees; Anchorage, Stockholm)

Time of Day	10 A.M.–12 P.M.				12 P.M.–3 P.M.				3 P.M.–5 P.M.			
Time of Year	Oct–Mar	Apr–May	Jun–Aug	Sep	Oct–Mar	Apr–May	Jun–Aug	Sep	Oct–Mar	Apr–May	Jun–Aug	Sep
Minutes of Sun												
Type 1 skin	0	20–25	15–20	20–25	0	10–20	5–10	10–20	0	20–25	15–20	20–25
Type 2 skin	0	25–40	20–30	25–40	0	15–25	10–15	15–25	0	25–40	20–30	25–40
Type 3 skin	0	30–50	25–40	30–50	0	20–30	15–20	20–30	0	30–50	25–40	30–50
Type 4 skin	0	45–60	30–50	45–60	0	30–40	20–30	30–40	0	45–60	30–50	45–60
Type 5–6 skin	0	60–90	50–60	60–90	0	40–60	30–40	40–60	0	60–90	50–60	60–90

Sunshine Is Powerful, All-Natural Medicine

Sunshine is not something to be irrationally feared. In fact, by now you should understand that there are numerous benefits associated with moderate exposure to UVB radiation. Thanks to the information in this chapter, you now have the precision tools to go out and get the right amount of sun to safely establish and maintain your vitamin D status and, in so doing, improve your health and prevent a variety of chronic diseases.

POSTSCRIPT

A S I WAS COMPLETING this book, an extraordinary amount of attention was being generated by an announcement concerning UV radiation and health. The federal government's National Toxicology Program had just come out with the statement that it had added ultraviolet radiation to the list of what it considers "known human carcinogens." As unfortunate as this move was by an agency of the U.S. Department of Health and Human Services, it perfectly encapsulates the misconceptions that prevail concerning sunlight and health, and it provides me with a final opportunity in this book to set the record straight.

The blanket statement that UV radiation is carcinogenic is confusing. As a friend of mine put it, saying that UV radiation causes cancer and should be avoided is akin to saying that water causes drowning, so don't drink water. It is misleading to place radiation on the list of carcinogens without saying that *overexposure* not just *exposure* is the problem.

The National Toxicology Program report, officially titled the *10th Report on Carcinogens*, was released in December 2002. The main problem with this report is that the criteria used to determine what substances would be listed don't take into consideration how much exposure you need for the substance to be harmful. Here is what the authors of the document themselves wrote when describing the criteria for selection: "The Report does not present quantitative assessments of carcinogenic risk. Listing of substances in the Report, therefore, does not establish that such substances present carcinogenic risks to individuals in their daily lives."

In my opinion, excluding this vital information makes the list of carcinogens pointless. The situation is similar to one in the 1980s, when the artificial sweetener *saccharine* was listed in the *Report on Carcinogens*. Remember those warning on the soda can labels stating that this product had been shown to cause cancer in laboratory animals? Significantly, saccharine was removed from the list in 2002 because the amount needed to cause cancer even in lab animals—800 cans of diet soda per rat!—was unrealistically large.

It's also important to keep in mind that carcinogens are present everywhere in nature. As scary as it may sound, there are known carcinogens in most food and drink, including tap water (chloroform), grain products (ethylene dibromide [EDB]), bacon and other processed meats (nitrosamines), peanut butter (aflatoxin), brown mustard (allylisothiocyanate), basil (estragole), mushrooms (hydrazines), beer and wine (ethyl alcohol), and as I just pointed out, some diet sodas (saccharine).

Here is what the American Council on Science and Health states about your chances of being free of all carcinogens: "No human diet can be free from all naturally occurring carcinogens or toxic substances. Indeed, it is hard to find *any* food that does not contain *some* harmful chemical that either occurs naturally

or is produced during cooking or by microbial decomposition."
The point I'm making is that carcinogens are everywhere—
including in natural substances that we need to survive. Just because something is natural doesn't mean we can consume or
subject ourselves to unlimited amounts of it without suffering
negative health consequences. Sugar, salt, and even oxygen are
all dangerous when taken in excess.

Interestingly, the rationale behind the decision to define
UV radiation as a carcinogen contradicts conclusions reached
about UV radiation by the U.S. Food and Drug Administration, which also happens to be part of the U.S. Department of
Health and Human Services. In a nutshell, the government is
disagreeing with itself.

Despite the attention the *10th Report on Carcinogens* received when UV radiation was put on its list of known human
carcinogens, the inclusion means nothing more than that overexposure to sunlight or a tanning bed may increase your risk
of skin cancer. There are few people around who would deny
this fact.

Clearly there's a lot of work to be done to promote the importance of UV radiation for all-around health. This book
should help alter public perception of the role of sunlight on
our lives. Certainly I hope it helps you make more informed
decisions about your relationship to sunshine, indoor tanning,
and human well-being.

Increasing numbers of scholarly articles are being published that address the beneficial relationship between UVB
radiation and good health. A major new article was published
in December 2002 in the official journal of the British Society
of Toxicology discussing the beneficial effects of sunlight on

the autoimmune diseases multiple sclerosis, Type 1 diabetes, and rheumatoid arthritis. This article explains how greater sun exposure was the reason certain populations had lower rates of these autoimmune diseases than people who had little sun exposure.

Sometimes great wisdom can be found in humor. When I came across a particular *Peanuts* cartoon by Charles Schultz, it occurred to me that what the legendary cartoonist had to say about sunshine really summed up everything I believe after more than thirty years in medicine (humbling as that might have been!). In the cartoon, Linus opens his lunch bag to find a note from his mom with a whole list of commonsense instructions for him. It concludes with this suggestion, "Are you sitting in the sun? I hope so, for a little sun is good as long as we don't overdo it. . . . Perhaps ten minutes a day this time of year is about right."

I couldn't have said it better myself.

GLOSSARY

actinic keratosis (pl. keratoses) This condition occurs as rough white, red, or brown scaly patches on the skin, usually in areas that have been exposed to the sun. Sometimes known as pre–skin cancer.

advanced sleep phase syndrome Disorder in which the major sleep episode is advanced in relation to the desired clock-time. Patients tend to feel groggy and tired in the afternoon, fall asleep in the early evening, and wake up in the middle of the night.

Alzheimer's disease Progressive, degenerative disease of the brain that causes impaired memory, thinking, and behavior.

apoptosis Mechanism that allows cells to self-destruct.

arthritis Inflammation of the joints often leading to their destruction. Acute arthritis is marked by pain, redness, and swelling.

basal cell Skin cell at the bottom of the epidermis that is constantly dividing and develops into the upper layers of the epidermis.

basal cell carcinoma This most common form of non-melanoma skin cancer affects the basal cells in the epidermis, causing them to reproduce uncontrollably. Usually occurs on areas of the skin that are most exposed to the sun.

beta endorphin The body's natural pain-killing hormone that is also responsible for certain feelings of well-being, sometimes referred to as a "natural high."

broad-spectrum sunscreen Sunscreen that protects against both UVA and UVB radiation.

cherry hemangioma Harmless, pinhead-sized cherry-red dome caused by a collection of dilated blood vessels.

circadian rhythm The cycle of changes people undergo every day that is regulated by our biological clocks.

cryosurgery Destruction by freezing with liquid nitrogen. A process used to remove or destroy skin cancers and other forms of cancer.

curettage Treatment that involves the use of a scalpel to cut out unwanted skin lesions, including some skin cancers.

delayed sleep phase syndrome Disorder in which the major sleep episode is delayed in relation to the desired clocktime. Patients find it difficult to fall asleep until the early hours of the morning.

dermis Inner layer of skin beneath the epidermis that contains blood vessels, lymph ducts, nerve fibers and nerve endings, hair follicles, sweat glands, and sebaceous glands, as well as the fibrous elastic network that provides cushion and support for the epidermis.

dysplastic nevi   Clusters of melanocytes and surrounding tissue, usually larger than a mole, with irregular and indistinct borders.

electrodesiccation   Treatment for skin cancer that involves using an electric needle to destroy tissue surrounding a removed section of skin.

epidemiologist   A scientist who investigates patterns of disease to find links between different factors.

epidermis   Outer layer of skin that is made up of basal and squamous cells, stratum corneum, and melanocytes.

erythema   Scientific term for the redness that can be caused by a sunburn.

fibromyalgia   Relatively new condition with symptoms of bone and muscle pain and weakness.

Holick Daily Value (HDV)   Recommended amount of vitamin D a person should receive. This amount is considerably larger than standard government recommendations.

hypertension   Condition that is the main cause of stroke and heart attacks. Also known as high blood pressure.

international unit (IU)   Quantity of a biologic substance (such as a vitamin) that produces a particular biological effect agreed upon as an international standard. For vitamin D, 1 IU equals 25 nanograms.

keratinocytes   Squamous cells of the epidermis.

laser surgery   Treatment for cancer that involves using a laser beam to cut away or vaporize growths.

lentigine   Flat brown patch with rounded edges that tends to occur on the skin of the face, hands, back, and feet. Also called liver spots or age spots.

lux   Measurement of light.

melanin   Pigment in the skin produced by the melanocytes that gives skin and hair its color.

melanocytes   Cells between the epidermis and dermis that produce melanin.

melanoma   Malignant tumor of the melanocytes.

melatonin   A hormone secreted by the pineal gland, especially in response to darkness, that causes drowsiness.

metastasize   Spread of cancer cells away from the original site of the disease, usually to other organs such as the lung, liver, brain, or lymph nodes.

minimal erythemal dose (1MED)   Length of time it takes a person to get a mild sunburn without sunscreen (pinkness to the skin).

multiple sclerosis (MS)   Chronic debilitating disease that affects the myelin sheath of brain and spinal cord nerves.

nevus (pl. nevi)   Pigmented area on the skin. Also known as mole or birthmark.

non-melanoma skin cancer Cancer of the basal or squamous cells.

osteomalacia Condition characterized by vague bone and muscle aches and weakness due to improper bone hardening. Sometimes called adult rickets.

osteoporosis Condition in which bones are riddled with holes and become porous, brittle, and weak, and therefore more susceptible to fractures.

p53 gene Gene responsible for making the p53 protein, whose function is to repair a damaged cell or cause it to kill itself.

photoaging Signs of aging in the skin caused or enhanced by the sun.

pineal gland A small gland in the brain that functions primarily as an endocrine organ to make melatonin and serotonin.

premenstrual syndrome (PMS) Group of symptoms that occurs regularly in conjunction with a woman's menstrual period.

psoralen UVA photochemotherapy (PUVA) Treatment of skin conditions that involves oral medications that make a patient's skin highly sensitive to UV radiation followed by carefully controlled exposure to sunlamps or natural sunlight.

rheumatoid arthritis (RA) Chronic inflammatory disease that primarily affects the joints but can also affect other organ systems.

rickets Condition in young children whose bones don't harden properly during development due to the lack of vitamin D, causing the bones to bend under the weight of the child's body. Also known as pediatric osteomalacia.

sclerosis Pathological hardening of tissue especially from overgrowth of fibrous tissue or increase in interstitial tissue.

seasonal affective disorder (SAD) Disorder that occurs with the changing seasons characterized by major depressive feelings during winter months.

seborrheic keratosis Wartlike, waxy-looking growth that appears to be pasted to the skin's surface and that may appear in a variety of colors.

sebum Oily substance created by sebaceous glands in the skin that helps prevent the skin from drying out.

serotonin A hormone produced by the pineal gland that makes people feel happy and alert. Also made elsewhere in the brain to act as a neurotransmitter.

shift worker's syndrome Condition suffered by people who work the night shift. Similar to SAD.

squamous cell Cells in the epidermis.

squamous cell carcinoma Type of skin cancer that occurs on areas that are most often exposed to extreme amounts of sun, such as the nose, top of the ears, and backs of the hands. Often appears as a firm red bump.

stratum corneum The very top layer of skin, which is made up of dead and peeling squamous cells that have been pushed toward the surface.

sunburn Inflamed, reddening of the skin subsequent to excessive UV exposure. The scientific term is erythema.

sun-phobe A person with an irrational fear of sunlight.

suprachiasmatic nucleus (SCN) Small cluster of cells located near the center of the brain that makes up our "biological clock."

synovium The membrane around a joint that makes a transparent viscid fluid to provide lubrication.

telangiectasias Collections of tiny red and blue blood vessels on the nose, chin, or cheeks that are a normal part of aging. May be caused by sun damage, liver disease, pregnancy, birth control pills, estrogen replacement therapy, or corticosteroids.

Type 1 diabetes Sometimes referred to as juvenile diabetes or insulin-dependant diabetes mellitus. This chronic disease occurs when the beta islet cells of the pancreas are attacked by the immune system and consequently don't produce enough insulin to regulate blood sugar levels.

ultraviolet (UV) radiation A form of electromagnetic radiation emitted by the sun.

UVA radiation Type of ultraviolet radiation with energies between 320 and 400 nanometers that reaches the earth. Causes wrinkles and may be responsible for melanomas.

UVB radiation   Type of ultraviolet radiation with energies between 290 and 319 nanometers that reaches the earth. Reddens the skin and can increase the risk of non-melanoma and melanoma skin cancers.

UVC radiation   Type of ultraviolet radiation with energies between 200 and 289 nanometers that is completely absorbed by earth's atmosphere.

vitamin D deficiency   Condition in which the body lacks enough vitamin D.

vitamin D toxicity   Condition in which the body has ingested too much vitamin D.

xeroderma pigmentosum (XP)   Extremely rare skin disorder in which a person is highly sensitive to sun exposure because of a genetic defect that prevents them from repairing even the most minor DNA damage from sun exposure.

BIBLIOGRAPHY

Aging Skin/Wrinkles

Contet-Audonneau, J.L., Jeanmaire, C., and Pauly, G. (1999). A histological study of human wrinkle structures: Comparison between sun-exposed areas of the face, with or without wrinkles, and sun-protected areas. *British Journal of Dermatology 140:* 1038–1047.

Holick, M.F., Ray, S., Chen, T., Tian, X., and Persons, K. (1994). Novel functions of a parathyroid hormone antagonist: Stimulation of epidermal proliferation and hair growth in mice. *Proceedings of the National Academy of Sciences 91:* 8014–8016.

Leung, W.C., and Harvey, I. (2002). Is skin ageing in the elderly caused by sun exposure or smoking? *British Journal of Dermatology 147*(6): 1187–1191.

Alzheimer's Disease

Ancoli-Israel, S., Martin, J.L., Kripke, D.F., Marler, M., and Klauber, M.R. (2002). Effect of light treatment on sleep and circadian rhythms in demented nursing home patients. *Journal of the American Geriatrics Society 50*(2): 282–289.

Campbell, S.S., et al. (1988). Exposure to light in healthy elderly subjects and Alzheimer's patients. *Physiology & Behavior 42*(2): 141–144.

Colenda, C.C., et al. (1997). Phototherapy for patients with Alzheimer disease with disturbed sleep patterns: Results of a community-based pilot study. *Alzheimer Disease and Associated Disorders 11*(3): 175–178.

Graf, A., et al. (2001). The effects of light therapy on mini-mental state examination scores in demented patients. *Biological Psychiatry 50*(9): 725–727.

Mishima, K., et al. (1994). Morning bright light therapy for sleep and behavior disorders in elderly patients with dementia. *Acta Psychiatrica Scandinavica 89*(1): 1–7.

Mishima, K., et al. (1998). Randomized, dim light controlled, crossover test of morning bright light therapy for rest-activity rhythm disorders in patients with vascular dementia and dementia of Alzheimer's type. *Chronobiology International 15*(6): 647–654.

Satlin, A., et al. (1992). Bright light treatment of behavioral and sleep disturbances in patients with Alzheimer's disease. *American Journal of Psychiatry 149*(8): 1028–1032.

Yamadera, H., et al. (2000). Effects of bright light on cognitive and sleep-wake (circadian) rhythm disturbances in Alzheimer-type dementia. *Psychiatry and Clinical Neurosciences 54*(3): 352–353.

Autoimmune Diseases (multiple sclerosis, rheumatoid arthritis, type 1 diabetes, etc.)

Ponsonby, A.-L., McMichael, A., and van der Mei, I. (2002). Ultraviolet radiation and autoimmune disease: Insights from epidemiological research. *Toxicology 181–182:* 71–78.

Cancer of the Internal Organs (breast, colon, ovaries, prostate, etc.)

Ahonen, M., Tenkanen, L., Teppo, L., Hakama, M., and Tuohimaa, P. (2000). Prostate cancer risk and prediagnostic serum 25-hydroxy-vitamin D levels. *Cancer Causes and Control 11:* 847–852.

Ainsleigh, H.G. (1993). Beneficial effects of sun exposure on cancer mortality. *Preventive Medicine 22*(1): 132–140.

Apperly, F.L. (1941). The relation of solar radiation to cancer mortality in North America. *Cancer Research 1:* 191–195.

Freedman, D.M., Dosemeci, M., and McGlynn, K. (2002). Sunlight and mortality from breast, ovarian, colon, prostate, and non-melanoma skin cancer: A composite death certificate based case-control study. *Occupational and Environmental Medicine 59*(4): 257–262.

Garland, C.F., Garland, F.C., Shaw, E.K., Comstock, G.W., Helsing, K.J., and Gorham, E.D. (1989). Serum 25-hydroxyvitamin D and colon cancer: Eight-year prospective study. *Lancet 18:* 1176–1178.

Garland, F.C., Garland, C.F., Gorham, E.D., and Young, J.F. (1990). Geographic variation in breast cancer mortality in the United States: A hypothesis involving exposure to solar radiation. *Preventive Medicine 19:* 614–622.

Grant, W.B. (2002). An ecologic study of dietary and solar ultraviolet-B links to breast carcinoma mortality rates. *Cancer 94*(1): 272–281.

Grant, W.B. (2002). An estimate of premature cancer mortality in the United States due to inadequate doses of solar ultraviolet-B radiation, a source of vitamin D. *Cancer 94*(6): 1867–1875.

Hanchette, C.L., and Schwartz, G.G. (1992). Geographic patterns of prostate cancer mortality: Evidence for a protective effect of ultraviolet radiation. *Cancer 70*(12): 2861–2869.

Havender, W.R. (1996). *Does Nature Know Best? Natural Carcinogens and Anticarcinogens in America's Food.* Originally written for the American Council on Science and Health. 5th Edition revised by Roger Coulombe, Ph.D., Professor of Toxicology and Molecular Biology and Director, Center for Environmental Toxicology at Utah State University.

Holick, M.F. (2001) Sunlight "dilemma": Risk of skin cancer or bone disease and muscle weakness. *Lancet 357*: 4–6.

John, E.M., Schwartz, G.G., Dreon, D.M., and Koo, J. (1999). Vitamin D and breast cancer risk: The NHANES I epidemiologic follow-up study, 1971–1975 to 1992. National Health and Nutrition Examination Survey. *Cancer Epidemiology, Biomarkers & Prevention 8(5)*: 399–406.

Lefkowitz, E.S., and Garland, C.F. (1994). Sunlight, vitamin D, and ovarian cancer mortality rates in U.S. women. *International Journal of Epidemiology 23(6)*: 1133–1136.

Luscombe, C.J., Fryer, A.A., French, M.E., Liu, S., Saxby, M.F., Jones, P.W., and Strange, R.C. (2001). Exposure to ultraviolet radiation: Association with susceptibility and age at presentation with prostate cancer. *Lancet 358(9282)*: 641–642.

National Toxicology Program, U.S. Department of Health and Human Services, Public Health Service. (2002). *10th Report on Carcinogens.* Pursuant to Section 301(b)(4) of the Public Health Service Act as Amended by Section 262, PL 95-622.

Schwartz, G.G., Whitlatch, L.W., Chen T.C., Lokeshwar, B.L., and Holick, M.F. (1998). Human prostate cells synthesize 1,25-dihydroxyvitamin D_3 from 25-hydroxyvitamin D_3. *Cancer Epidemiology, Biomarkers & Prevention 7*: 391–395.

Tangpricha, V., Flanagan, J.N., Whitlatch, L.W., Tseng, C.C., Chen, T.C., Holt, P.R., Lipkin, M.S., and Holick, M.F. (2001). 25-hydroxyvitamin D-1[alpha]-hydroxylase in normal and malignant colon tissue. *Lancet 357*: 1673–1674.

Cardiovascular Health

Holick, M.F. (2002). Sunlight and vitamin D: Both good for cardiovascular health. *Journal of General Internal Medicine 17*: 733–735.

Krause, R., Buhring, M., Hopfenmuller, W., Holick, M.F., and Sharma, A.M. (1998). Ultraviolet B and blood pressure. *Lancet 352*(9129): 709–710.

Li, Y., Kong, J., Wei, M., Chen, Z.F., Liu, S., and Cao, L.P. (2002). 1,25-dihydroxyvitamin D_3 is a negative endocrine regulator of the renin-angiotensin system. *Journal of Clinical Investigation 110*(2): 229–238.

Rostand, S.G. (1979). Ultraviolet light may contribute to geographic and racial blood pressure differences. *Hypertension 30*: 150–156.

Scragg, R., Jackson, R., Holdaway, I.M., Lim, T., and Beaglehole, R. (1990). Myocardial infarction is inversely associated with plasma 25-hydroxyvitamin D_3 levels: A community-based study. *International Journal of Epidemiology 19*: 559–563.

Zitterman, A., Schulze Schleithoff, S., Tenderich, C., Berthold, H., Koefer, R., and Stehle, P. (2003). Low vitamin D status: A contributing factor in the pathogenesis of congestive heart failure? *Journal of the American College of Cardiology 41*(1): 105–112.

Circadian Rhythms

Ancoli-Israel, S., Martin, J.L., Kripke, D.F., Marler, M., and Klauber, M.R. (2002). Effect of light treatment on sleep and circadian rhythms in demented nursing home patients. *Journal of the American Geriatrics Society 50*(2): 282–289.

Brainard, G.C., Hanifin, J.P., Rollag, M.D., Greeson, J., Byrne, B., Glick-man, G., Gerner, E., and Sanford, B. (2001). Human melatonin reg-ulation is not mediated by the three cone photopic visual system. *Journal of Clinical Endocrinology and Metabolism 86*(1): 433–436.

Campbell, S.S., and Murphy, P.J. (1998). Extraocular circadian photo-transduction in humans. *Chronobiology International 279*: 396–399.

Czeisler, C.A., et al. (1995). Use of bright light to treat maladaptation to night shift work and circadian rhythm sleep disorders. *Journal of Sleep Research 4*(S2): 70–73.

Czeisler, C.A., Shanahan, T.L., Klerman, E.B., Martens, H., Brotman, D.J., Emens, J.S., Klein, T., and Rizzo, J.F. (1995). Suppression of melatonin secretion in some blind patients by exposure to bright light. *New England Journal of Medicine 332*: 6–11.

Eastman, C.I., et al. (1999). How to use light and dark to produce circa-dian adaptation to night shift work. *Annals of Medicine 31*(2): 87–98.

Midwinter, M.J., et al. (1991). Adaptation of the melatonin rhythm in human subjects following night-shift work in Antarctica. *Neuroscience Letters 122*(2): 195–198.

Zanello, S.B., Jackson, D., and Holick, M.F. (2000). Expression of the cir-cadian clock genes *clock* and *period 1* in human skin. *Journal of Inves-tigative Dermatology 115*(4): 757–760.

Depression: Seasonal and Nonseasonal

Czeisler, C.A., et al. (1995). Use of bright light to treat maladaptation to night shift work and circadian rhythm sleep disorders. *Journal of Sleep Research 4*(S2): 70–73.

Eastman, C.I., et al. (1998). Bright light treatment of winter depression. *Archives of General Psychiatry 55*: 883–889.

Gambichler, T, et al. (2002). Impact of UVA exposure on psychological parameters and circulating serotonin and melatonin. *Dermatology* 2(1): 6.

Gloth, F.M., Alam, W., and Hollis, B. (1999). Vitamin D vs broad spectrum phototherapy in the treatment of seasonal affective disorder. *The Journal of Nutrition, Health and Aging 3:* 5–7.

Kripke, D.F. (1998). Light treatment for nonseasonal depression: Speed, efficacy, and combined treatment. *Journal of Affective Disorders 49*(2): 109–117.

Kripke, D.F., Risch, S.C., and Janowsky, D. (1983). Bright white light alleviates depression. *Psychiatry Research 10*(2): 105–112.

Lam, R.W., et al. (1989). Phototherapy for depressive disorders: A review. *Canadian Journal of Psychiatry 34*(2): 140–147.

Lam, R.W., and Levitt, A.J. (eds.). (2000). Canadian consensus guidelines for the treatment of seasonal affective disorder: A summary of the report of the Canadian consensus group on SAD. *Canadian Journal of Diagnosis.*

Levins, P.C., Carr, D.B., Fisher, J.E., Momtaz, K., and Parrish, J.A. (1983). Plasma [beta]-endorphin and [beta]-lipotropin response to ultraviolet radiation. *Lancet* 2(8342): 166.

Lewy, A.J., et al. (1998). Morning vs. evening light treatment of patients with winter depression. *Archives of General Psychiatry 55:* 890–896.

Loving, R.T., Kripke, D.F., and Shuchter, S.R. (2002). Bright light augments antidepressant effects of medication and wake therapy. *Depression and Anxiety 16*(1): 1–3.

Partonen, T., and Lonnqvist, J. (1998). Seasonal affective disorder. *Lancet 352:* 1369–1374.

Pinchasov, B.B., et al. (2002). Mood and energy regulation in seasonal and non-seasonal depression before and after midday treatment with physical exercise or bright light. *Psychiatry Research 94*(1): 29–42.

Prasko, J., et al. (2002). Bright light therapy and/or imipramine for inpatients with recurrent non-seasonal depression. *Neuroendocrinology Letters 23*(2): 109–113.

Rao, M.L., et al. (1990). The influence of phototherapy on serotonin and melatonin in non-seasonal depression. *Pharmacopsychiatry 23*(3): 155–158.

Rosenthal, N.E. (1993). Diagnosis and treatment of seasonal affective disorder. *Journal of the American Medical Association 270*(22): 2717–2720.

Rosenthal, N.E., Sack, D.A., Gillin, J.C., Lewy, A.J., Goodwin, F.K., Davenport, Y., Mueller, P.S., Newsome, D.A., and Wehr, T.A. (1984). Seasonal affective disorder: A description of the syndrome and preliminary findings with light therapy. *Archives of General Psychiatry 41*(1): 72–80.

Swartz, P.J., et al. (1996). Winter seasonal affective disorder: A follow-up study of the first 59 patients of the National Institute of Mental Health Seasonal Studies Program. *American Journal of Psychiatry 153*(8): 1028–1036.

Terman, M., et al. (1998). A controlled trial of timed bright light and negative air ionization for treatment of winter depression. *Archives of General Psychiatry 55*: 875–882.

Wetterberg, L. (1992). Light therapy of depression; basal and clinical aspects. *Pharmacology & Toxicology 71*(Suppl 1): 96–106.

Wurtman, R.J., and Wurtman, J.J. (1989). Carbohydrates and depression. *Scientific American 260*: 68–75.

Diabetes (see also Autoimmune Diseases)

Hypponen, E., Laara, E., Reunanen, A., Jarvelin, M.R., and Virtanen, S.M. (2001). Intake of vitamin D and risk of type 1 diabetes: A birth-cohort study. *Lancet 358*(9292): 1500–1503.

Mathieu, C., Waer, M., Laureys, J., Rutgeerts, O., and Bouillon, R. (1994). Prevention of autoimmune diabetes in NOD mice by 1,25 dihydroxyvitamin D₃. *Diabetologia 37:* 552–558.

Norris, J.M. (2001). Can the sunshine vitamin shed light on type 1 diabetes? *Lancet 358*(9292): 1476–1478.

Multiple Sclerosis (see also Autoimmune Diseases)

Cantorna, M.T., Hayes, C.E., and DeLuca, H.F. (1996). 1,25-Dihydroxy-vitamin D₃ reversibly blocks the progression of relapsing encephalomyelitis, a model of multiple sclerosis. *Proceedings of the National Academy of Sciences 93:* 7861–7864.

Hayes, C., Cantorna, M.T., Deluca, H.F. (1997). Vitamin D and multiple sclerosis. *Proceedings of the Society for Experimental Biology and Medicine 216:* 21–27.

Hernan, M.A., Olek, M.J., Ascherio, A. (1999). Geographic variation of MS incidence in two prospective studies of US women. *Neurology 51:* 1711–1718.

Hogancamp, W.E., Rodriguez, M., Weinshenker, B.G. (1997). The epidemiology of multiple sclerosis. *Mayo Clinic Proceedings 72:* 871–878.

Obesity

Wortsman, J., Matsuoka, L.Y., Chen, T.C., Lu, Z., and Holick, M.F. (2000). Decreased bioavailability of vitamin D in obesity. *American Journal of Clinical Nutrition 72*(3): 690–693.

Osteomalacia/Fibromyalgia

Glerup, H., and Eriksen, E. (2001). Hypovitaminosis D myopathy. In M.F. Holick (ed.), *Biological Effects of Light* (pp. 185–192). Boston: Kluwer Academic Publishers.

Malabanan, A.O., Turner, A.K., and Holick, M.F. (1998). Severe general-ized bone pain and osteoporosis in a premenopausal black female: Effect of vitamin D replacement. *Journal of Clinical Densitometry 1:* 201–204.

Osteoporosis

Chapuy, M.C., Arlot, M.E., Duboeuf, F., et al. (1992). Vitamin D_3 and calcium to prevent hip fractures in elderly women. *New England Journal of Medicine 327:* 1637–1642.

Dawson-Hughes, B., Harris, S.S., Krall, E.A., and Dallal, G.E. (1997). Effect of calcium and vitamin D supplementation on bone density in men and women 65 years of age or older. *New England Journal of Medicine 337:* 670–676.

Heikinheimo, R.J., Inkovaara, J.A., Harju, E.J., Haavisto, M.V., Kaarela, R.H., Kataja, J.M., Kokko, A.M., Kolho, L.A., and Rajala, S.A. (1992). Annual injection of vitamin D and fractures of aged bones. *Calcified Tissue International 51*(2): 105–110.

Rosen, C.J., Morrison, A., Zhou, H., Storm, D., Hunter, S.J., Musgrave, K., Chen, T., Wen-Wei, L., and Holick, M.F. (1994). Elderly women in northern New England exhibit seasonal changes in bone mineral density and calciotropic hormones. *Bone and Mineral 25:* 83–92.

Premenstrual Syndrome

Anderson, D.J., Legg, N.J., and Ridout, D.A. (1997). Preliminary trial of photic stimulation for premenstrual syndrome. *Journal of Obstetrics and Gynaecology 17*(1): 76–79.

Lam, R.W., et al. (1999). A controlled study of light therapy in women with late luteal phase dysphoric disorder. *Psychiatry Research 86*(3): 185–192.

Parry, B.L., et al. (1987). Treatment of a patient with seasonal premenstrual syndrome. *American Journal of Psychiatry 144*(6): 762–766.

Parry, B.L., et al. (1989). Morning versus evening bright light treatment of late luteal phase dysphoric disorder. *American Journal of Psychiatry 146*(9): 1215–1217.

Parry, B.L., et al. (1991). Atenolol in premenstrual syndrome: A test of the melatonin hypothesis. *Psychiatry Research 37*(2): 131–138.

Parry, B.L., et al. (1997). Blunted phase-shift responses to morning bright light in premenstrual dysphoric disorder. *Journal of Biological Rhythms 12*(5): 443–456.

Psoriasis

Diffey, B.L., Larko, O., and Swanbeck, G. (1981). UV-B doses received during different outdoor activities and UV-B treatment of psoriasis. *British Journal of Dermatology 106:* 33–41.

Holick, M.F. (1998). Clinical efficacy of 1,25dihydroxyvitamin D_3 and its analogues in the treatment of psoriasis. *Retinoids 14*(1): 12–17.

Nickoloff, B., Schroder, J., von den Driesch, P., Raychaudhuri, S., Farber, E., Boehncke, W.-H., Morhenn, V., Rosenberg, E., Schon, M., and Holick, M.F. (2000). Is psoriasis a T-cell disease? *Experimental Dermatology 9:* 359–375.

Perez, A., Chen, T.C., Turner, A., Raab, R., Bhawan, J., Poche, P., and Holick, M.F. (1996). Efficacy and safety of topical calcitriol (1,25-dihydroxyvitamin D₃) for the treatment of psoriasis. *British Journal of Dermatology 134:* 238–246.

Rheumatoid Arthritis (see also Autoimmune Diseases)

Cantorna, M.T., Hayes, C.E., and DeLuca, H.F. (1998). 1,25-Dihydroxy-cholecalciferol inhibits the progression of arthritis in murine models of human arthritis. *Journal of Nutrition 128:* 68–72.

Rickets

Hess, A.F., and Unger, L.F. (1921). Cure of infantile rickets by sunlight. *Journal of the American Medical Association 77:* 33–41.

Kreiter, S.R., Schwartz, R.P., Kirkman, H.N., Charlton, P.A., Calikoglu, A.S., and Davenport, M. (2000). Nutritional rickets in African American breast-fed infants. *Journal of Pediatrics 137:* 2–6.

Opp, T.E. (1964). Infantile hypercalcaemia, nutritional rickets, and infantile scurvy in Great Britain. *British Medical Journal 1:* 1659–1661.

Sniadecki, J. (1840). *On the Cure of Rickets.* Cited by W. Mozolowski in *Nature 143:* 141 (1939).

Skin Cancer

Black H, et al. (1995). Evidence that a low-fat diet reduces the occurrence of non-melanoma skin cancer. *International Journal of Cancer 62(2):* 165–169.

Garland, F.C., and Garland, C.F. (1990). Occupational sunlight exposure and melanoma in the U.S. Navy. *Archives of Environmental Health 45* (5): 261–267.

Ziegler, A., Jonason, A.S., Leffell, D.J., Simon, J.A., Sharma, H.W., Kimmelman, J., Remington, L., Jacks, T., and Brash, D.E. (1994). Sunburn and p53 in the onset of skin cancer. *Nature 372:* 773–776.

Sleep Disorders

Terman, M., Lewy, A.J., Dijk, D.-J., Boulos, Z., Eastman, C.I., and Campbell, S.S. (1995). Light treatment for sleep disorders: Consensus report. IV. Sleep phase and duration disturbances. *Journal of Biological Rhythms 10:* 135–147.

Tanning Bed Therapy

Koutkia, P., Lu, Z., Chen, T.C., and Holick, M.F. (2001). Treatment of vitamin D deficiency due to Crohn's disease with tanning bed ultraviolet B radiation. *Gastroenterology 121:* 1485–1488.

Vitamin D Deficiency

Chapuy, M.C., Arlot, M., Duboeuf, F., Brun, J., Crouzet, B., Arnaud, S., Delmas, P., and Meunier, P.J. (1992). Vitamin D_3 and calcium to prevent hip fractures in elderly women. *New England Journal of Medicine 327:* 1627–1642.

Chapuy, M.C., Preziosi, P., Maaner, M., Arnaud, S., Galan, P., Hercberg, S., and Meunier, P.J. (1997). Prevalence of vitamin D insufficiency in an adult normal population. *Osteoporosis International 7:* 439–443.

Glerup, H., Middelsen, K., Poulsen, L., Hass, E., Overbeck, S., Andersen, H., Charles, P., and Eriksen, E.F. (2000). Hypovitaminosis D myopathy without biochemical signs of osteomalacia bone involvement. *Calcified Tissue International 66:* 419–424.

Holick, M.F. (2002). Too little vitamin D in pre-menopausal women: Why should we care? *American Journal of Clinical Nutrition 76:* 3–4.

Holick, M.F. (2002). Vitamin D: The underappreciated D-lightful hormone that is important for skeletal and cellular health. *Current Opinion on Endocrinology and Diabetes 9:* 87–98.

Malabanan, A., Veronikis, I.E., and Holick, M.F. (1998). Redefining vitamin D insufficiency. *Lancet 351:* 805–806.

Nesby-O'Dell, S., Scanlon, K., Cogswell, M., Gillespie, C., Hollis, B., and Looker, A. (2002). Hypovitaminosis D prevalence and determinants among African American and white women of reproductive age: Third national health and nutrition examination survey, 1988–1994. *American Journal of Clinical Nutrition 76:* 187–192.

Tangpricha, V., Pearce, E.N., Chen, T.C., and Holick, M.F. (2002). Vitamin D insufficiency among free-living healthy young adults. *American Journal of Medicine 112:* 659–662.

Vitamin D in Milk and Orange Juice

Holick, M.F., Shao, Q., Liu, W.W., and Chen, T.C. (1992). The vitamin D content of fortified milk and infant formula. *New England Journal of Medicine 326:* 1178–1181.

Tangpricha, V., Koutkia, P., Rieke, S.M., Chen, T.C., Perez, A.A., and Holick, M.F. Fortification of orange juice with vitamin D: A novel approach to enhance vitamin D nutritional health. *American Journal of Clinical Nutrition.* In press.

Vitamin D Nutrition

Barger-Lux, M.J., Heaney, R.P., Dowell, S., Chen, T.C., and Holick, M.F. (1998). Vitamin D and its major metabolites: Serum levels after graded oral dosing in healthy men. *Osteoporosis International 8:* 222–230.

Dawson-Hughes, B., Harris, S.S., and Dallal, G.E. (1997). Plasma calcidiol, season, and serum parathyroid hormone concentrations in healthy elderly men and women. *American Journal of Clinical Nutrition 65:* 67–71.

Heaney, R.P., Barger-Lux, J., Dowell, M.S., Chen, T.C., and Holick, M.F. (1997). Calcium absorptive effects of vitamin D and its major metabolites. *Journal of Clinical Endocrinology and Metabolism 82:* 4111–4116.

Holick, M.F. (1998). Vitamin D requirements for humans of all ages: New increased requirements for women and men 50 years and older. *Osteoporosis International 8:* S24–S29.

Vieth, R., Chan, P.C., and MacFarlane, G.D. (2001). Efficacy and safety of vitamin D_3 intake exceeding the lowest observed adverse effect level. *American Journal of Clinical Nutrition 73:* 288–294.

Vitamin D Skin Synthesis

Chel, V.G.M., Ooms, M.E., Popp-Snijders, C., Pavel, S., Schothorst, A.A., Meulemans, C.C.E., and Lips, P. (1998). Ultraviolet irradiation corrects vitamin D deficiency and suppresses secondary hyperparathyroidism in the elderly. *Journal of Bone and Mineral Research 13:* 1238–1242.

Chuck, A., Todd, J., and Diffey, B. (2001). Subliminal ultraviolet-B irradiation for the prevention of vitamin D deficiency in the elderly: A feasibility study. *Photodermatology, Photoimmunology and Photomedicine* *17*(4): 168–171.

Haddad, J.G., Matsuoka, L.Y., Hollis, B.W., Hu, Y.Z., and Wortsman, J. (1993). Human plasma transport of vitamin D after its endogenous synthesis. *Journal of Clinical Investigation 91:* 2552–2555.

Holick, M.F. (2003). Vitamin D: A millennium perspective. *Journal of Cellular Biochemistry 88:* 296–307.

Matsuoka, L.Y., Ide, L., Wortsman, J., MacLaughlin, J., and Holick, M.F. (1987). Sunscreens suppress cutaneous vitamin D_3 synthesis. *Journal of Clinical Endocrinology and Metabolism 64:* 1165–1168.

Matsuoka, L.Y., Wortsman, J., Hanifan, N., and Holick, M.F. (1988). Chronic sunscreen use decreases circulating concentrations of 25-hydroxyvitamin D: A preliminary study. *Archives of Dermatology 124:* 1802–1804.

Matsuoka, L.Y., Wortsman, J., Dannenberg, M.J., Hollis, B.W., Lu, Z., and Holick, M. F. (1992). Clothing prevents ultraviolet-B radiation-dependent photosynthesis of vitamin D_3. *Journal of Clinical Endocrinology and Metabolism 75:* 1099–1103.

Matsuoka, L.Y., McConnachie, P., Wortsman, J., and Holick, M.F. (1999). Immunological responses to ultraviolet light B radiation in black individuals. *Life Sciences 64:* 1563–1569.

Tian, X.Q., Chen, T.C., Matsuoka, L.Y., Wortsman, J., and Holick, M.F. (1993). Kinetic and thermodynamic studies of the conversion of previtamin D_3 to vitamin D_3 in human skin. *Journal of Biological Chemistry 268:* 14888–14892.

Webb, A.R., Pilbeam, C., Hanafin, N., and Holick, M.F. (1990). A one-year study to evaluate the roles of exposure to sunlight and diet on the circulating concentrations of 25-OH-D in an elderly population in Boston. *American Journal of Clinical Nutrition 51:* 1075–1081.

Webb, A.R., Kline, L., and Holick, M.F. (1998). Influence of season and latitude on the cutaneous synthesis of vitamin D_3: Exposure to winter sunlight in Boston and Edmonton will not promote vitamin D_3 synthesis in human skin. *Journal of Clinical Endocrinology and Metabolism* 67: 373–378.

Books

Holick, M.F. (ed.). (1998). *Vitamin D: Physiology, Molecular Biology, and Clinical Applications.* Totowa, NJ: Humana Press.

Holick, M.F. (ed.). (2001). *Biologic Effects of Light* (Proceedings of Symposium, Boston, MA). Boston: Kluwer Academic Publishing.

Holick, M.F., and Kligman, A. (eds.). (1992). *Biologic Effects of Light* (Proceedings of Symposium, Atlanta, GA). Berlin: Walter de Gruyter.

Holick, M.F., and Jung, E.G. (eds.). (1996). *Biologic Effects of Light* (Proceedings of Symposium, Atlanta, GA). Berlin: Walter de Gruyter.

Holick, M.F., and Jung, E.G. (eds.). (1999). *Biologic Effects of Light* (Proceedings of Symposium, Basel, Switzerland). Boston: Kluwer Academic Publishing.

Jung, E.G., and Holick, M.F. (eds.). (1994). *Biologic Effects of Light* (Proceedings of Symposium, Basel, Switzerland). Berlin: Walter de Gruyter.

INDEX

ABOUT THE
AUTHORS

Michael F. Holick, Ph.D., M.D., is internationally recognized for his expertise and many contributions in the fields of vitamin D, calcium, skin, bone, and the biologic effects of light. At Boston University School of Medicine, Dr. Holick is professor of medicine, dermatology, and physiology and biophysics; director of the Bone Health Care Clinic; and program director of the General Clinical Research Center. Dr. Holick was a merit awardee of the National Institutes of Health, serves as Chairman of a Review Group for NASA, and has served on the editorial boards of major journals. He has published more than two hundred articles in respected scientific journals and has been the chair and co-chair for the biannual Symposium on the Biologic Effects of Light for the past decade. Dr. Holick is a member of numerous prestigious academic associations and has received more than forty awards and honors for his innovative research and clinical activities, including the 2003 Robert H. Herman Award from the American Society of Clinical Nutrition. Dr. Holick's Vitamin D, Skin, and Bone research laboratory at the Boston University School of Medicine emphasizes the development of new approaches for treating osteoporosis, skin diseases, and cancer of the skin, breast, colon, and prostate.

Dr. Holick lives in Sudbury, Massachusetts, with his wife Sally and daughter and can be found working in the garden or on the tennis court.

Mark Jenkins is the author and co-author of a dozen books, including two Book-of-the-Month Club alternate selections. His writing has appeared in publications as varied as *Rolling Stone* and *The Wall Street Journal*. Mr. Jenkins also writes humorous commentaries for public radio about life on a small island. He lives on the island of Martha's Vineyard with his partner Patty and her two sons, where he enjoys bodysurfing and tennis.

For sales, editorial information, subsidiary rights information
or a catalog, please write or phone or e-mail

ibooks
1230 Park Avenue
New York, New York 10128, US
Sales: 1-800-68-BRICK
Tel: 212-427-7139 Fax: 212-860-8852
www.ibooksinc.com
email: bricktower@aol.com.

For sales in the United States, please contact
National Book Network
nbnbooks.com
Orders: 800-462-6420
Fax: 800-338-4550
custserv@nbnbooks.com

For sales in the UK and Europe please contact our distributor,
Gazelle Book Services
Falcon House, Queens Square
Lancaster, LA1 1RN, UK
Tel: (01524) 68765 Fax: (01524) 63232
email: gazelle4go@aol.com.

For Australian and New Zealand sales please contact
Bookwise International
174 Cormack Road, Wingfield, 5013, South Australia
Tel: 61 (0) 419 340056 Fax: 61 (0)8 8268 1010
email: karen.emmerson@bookwise.com.au